THE MAGIC OF AFRICA

Maria Bárkányi Csávás

Over one million people each year commit suicide
- World Health organization

All rights reserved, no part of this publication may be reproduced by any means, electronic, mechanical, or photocopying, documentary, film, or otherwise without prior permission of the publisher.

Published by:
Chipmunkapublishing Ltd
PO Box 6872
Brentwood
Essex
CM13 1ZT
United Kingdom

http://www.chipmunkapublishing.com
Chipmunkapublishing is dedicated to raising awareness of all mental health issues and facts

Copyright © 2007 Maria Bárkányi Csávás

All rights reserved
Photographs or text contained in this book may not be used without the consent of the author.

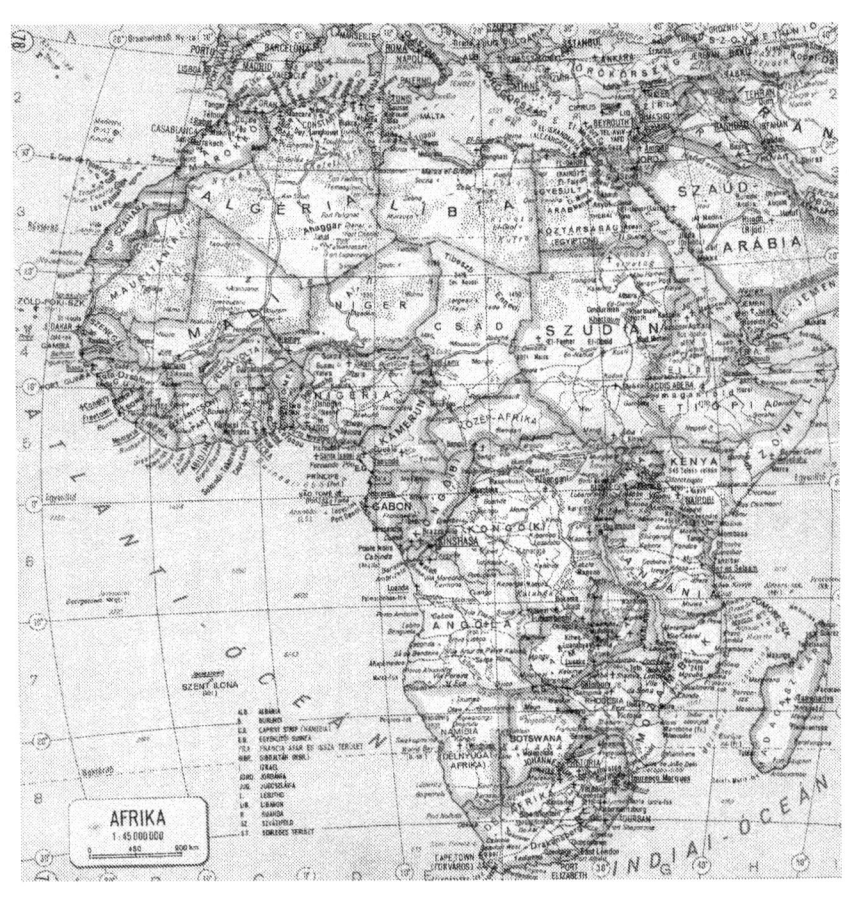

The map of Africa

Contents

Introduction
The Magic of Africa
West-Africa
BENIN (Dahomey)
    The Voodoo Cult
NIGERIA
    The countryside
    Everyday life
    Deep in the bush
    Markets
    Culture & Folk art
    Body adornment, Scar tattoo, Dance
    Sallah Festival
East-Africa
THE SUDAN
    The Sahel- zone
    Darfur province
DISEASE
THE VOICE OF AFRICA
KENYA
    The Eden of Africa
Conclusion

Introduction

Over a period of ten years from 1980-1990, we travelled the vast and wonderful continent of Africa.
The photographs contained in this book were taken by my husband, who worked in the Sudan and Nigeria as an FAO agricultural adviser.
The pictures are snapshot images of Niger, Benin, Nigeria, the Sudan [Darfur] through to Kenya. We didn't visit all the countries of Africa, but those which we did represent a good cross- section.
This book is intended to provide general information as well as our impressions of these countries.
It is impossible not to speak about the major problems facing Africa, such as famine, lack of consensus, birth control, disease, and lack of clean water. So I will touch a bit upon this too.
I know that the photographs and my memories of Africa are from some time ago and many things have surely changed by now, but the major problems are still there.

The aim of this book is to raise public awareness in the developed countries of the world and prompt them to provide more help to Africa.
Africa is not just a safari. There are many people dying of hunger. This is a continent blessed with extraordinary beauty and one which deserves the practical assistance of the developed world.
Our dream? To help Africa a little in our own small way by offering the royalties of this book to a charity organisation.

If you have bought this book, you have already helped Africa too.

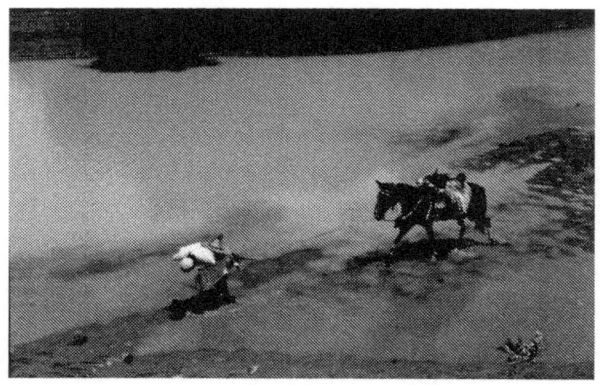

Picture 1: Kuzuntu – Nigeria.
Shallows on the river Kuzuntu.

Magic of Africa

Although you can leave Africa, you can never leave it behind and you can never forget it. I can still feel its dusty taste in my mouth as we roamed endlessly. Great journeys and conquering huge distances have always been part of our life. Many times, we fought with the bogged down land rover on untrodden paths in the bush. We fought mosquitoes, heat and dust. It wasn't easy. But our interest in Africa and our great love of the continent kept us going.

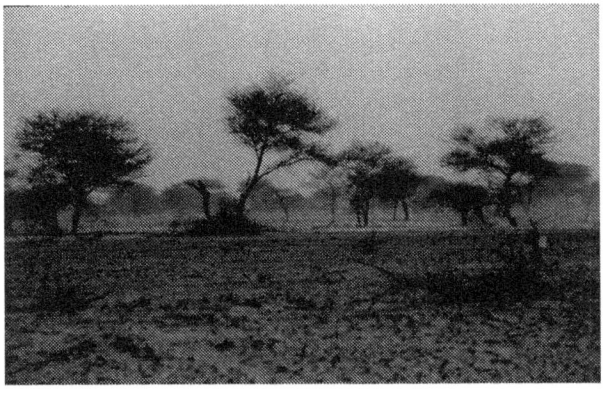

Picture 2 : North of Nigeria. Harmattan [dust wind] in the savannah.

I still remember catching sight of the assembled crowd of different nomadic tribes [who live in the semi-desert] in the Sunday market. It was like a scene from the tales of Sheherezade. Their black, indigo blue, light blue and white long dresses, which covered the whole body, the different shape of turbans, the beautiful handmade weapons, knives, bags, the strange smell of spices and the colourful ornaments create an exotic impression.

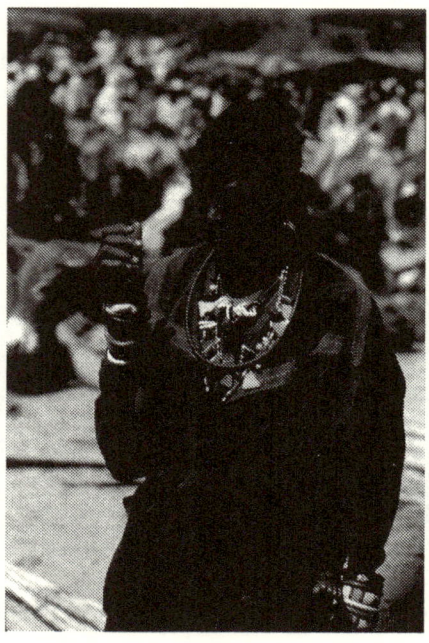

Picture   3:   South of Niger. In the Sunday market. Multi-coloured beads and bracelets are a popular decorative element all over Africa.

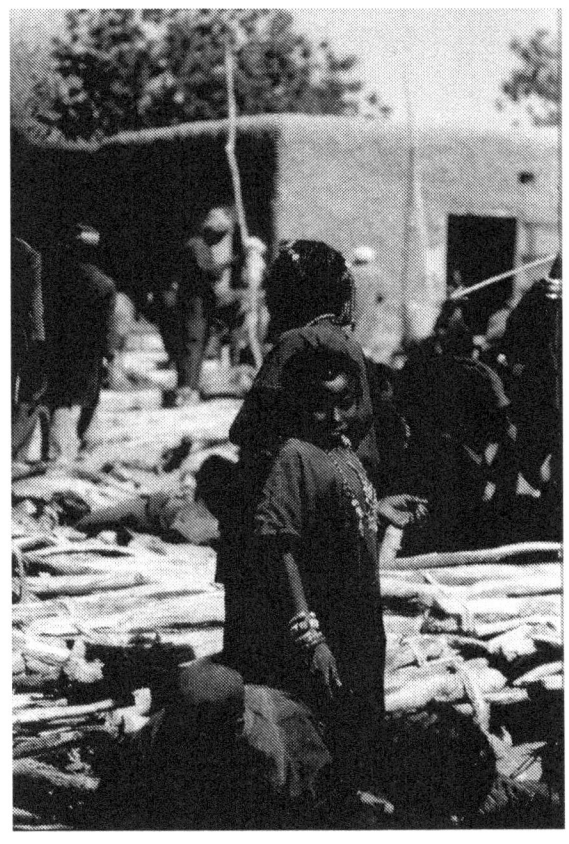

Picture 4: South of Niger. Firewood sellers.

At the edge of the Sahara, firewood is rather expensive because everybody cooks on an open fire in the countryside.

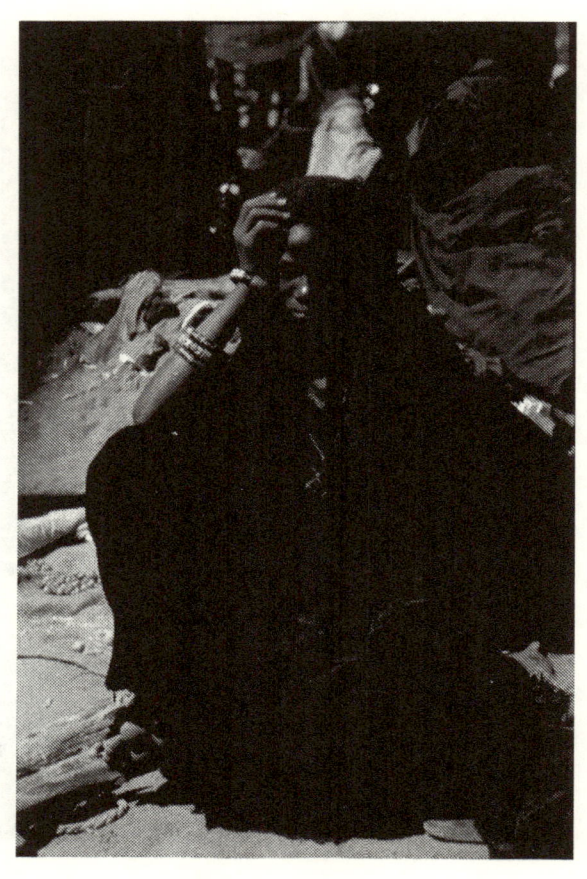

Picture 5: South of Niger.

In the market.
Tuareg woman in indigo blue clothes.

During our various travels, we saw beyond the glitter of the big cities to the poverty of the homeless. We often saw villages hidden in the bush where people worked very hard for their simple life.

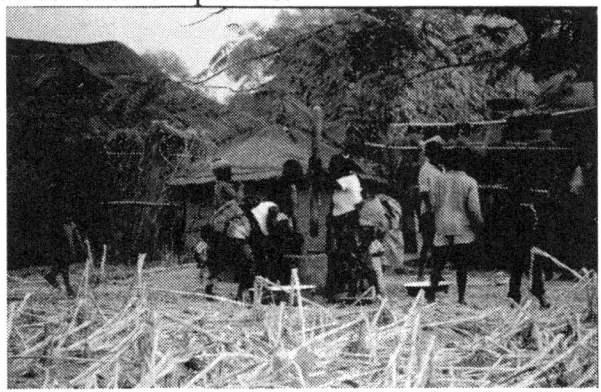

Picture 6: North – Nigeria. Everyday life in a small village.

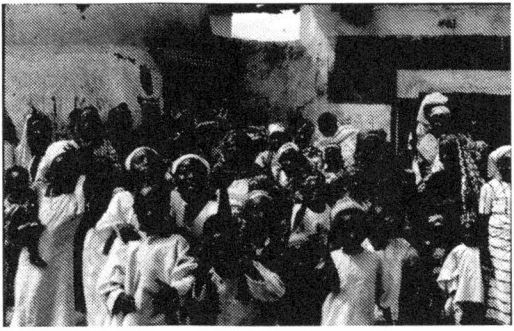

Picture 7: Nigeria –Zaria. On a festival or any celebration day, the people are happy, singing and

dancing, and for a short time they are able forget their daily life.

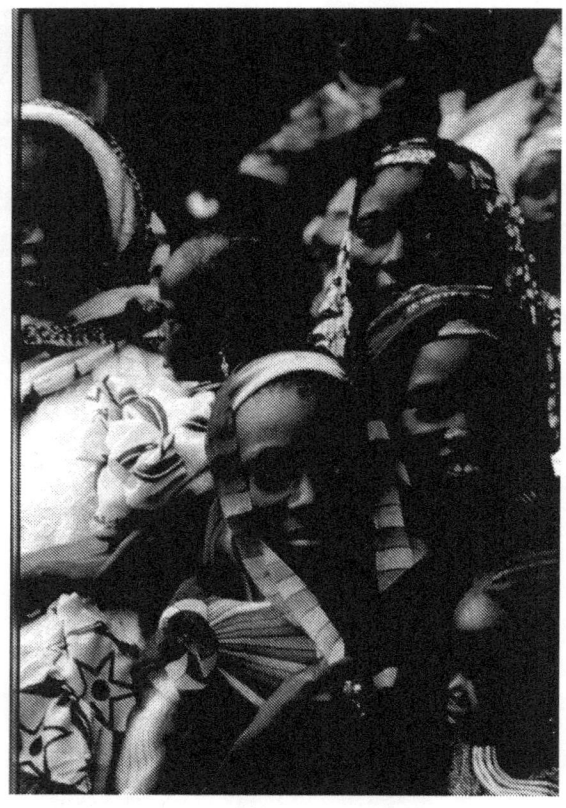

Picture   8:   Nigeria – Zaria. Hausa girls.

And as I walked in the heart of the savannah, I was seized by feeling of wonder at these vast areas, where

the harmony of the colours radiates tranquillity on motionless land.
Such magic often touched me. The beauty of nature blended with the calmness and peace of life.

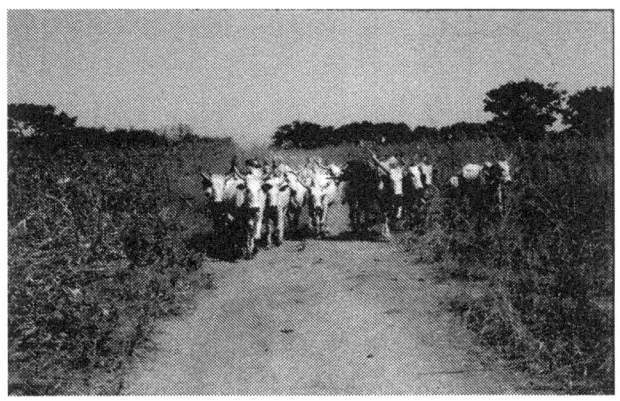

Picture   9:   North - Nigeria.   The herd together.

In the distance, through the tremble of hot air, nomads came closer and closer and behind them, the dust cloud of the herd turned gold in the last rays of the sun. The herd stopped and settled and it was not long before smoke was rising into the sky as darkness covered the savannah. The small fire was the only indication of life.

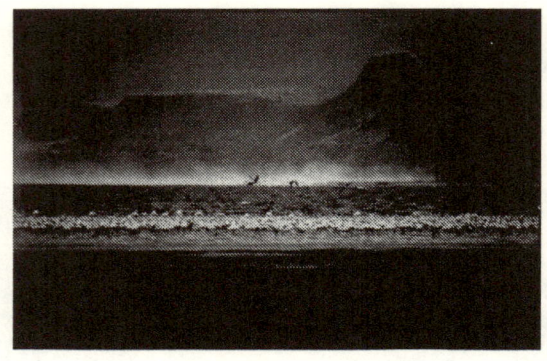

Picture 10: Lake Nakuru - Kenya. It is a place I will remember forever.

West - Africa

BENIN [Dahomey]

Until 1980, Dahomey was a French colony. On gaining independence, its name was changed to Benin. This is a country with a population of barely six million, where living standards are very low. The average life span is only 41 years.
Almost the entire country is covered by savannah. Forests are few, arable land is poor. The basic agricultural activities are mostly palm oil and cotton production.
The larger ethnic groups are the Fon, Somba [Bariba], Yoruba and the Tofin.

Our first visit was to the village of the friendly Tofin, near Cotonou. Ganvie village is full of wooden huts which are built on tall poles on the Nakoue lagoon. This makes the village unique in the whole of West Africa. In the middle of the 18th century, the Tofins escaped an attack by the Fons and managed to flee as far as the middle of the lagoon, where they set up a village.

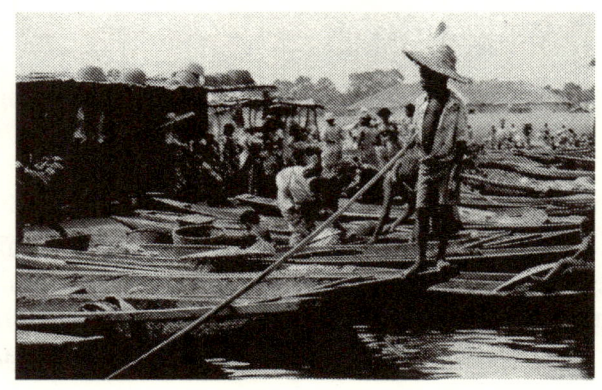

Picture   11:   Nakoue lagoon.

The only means of transport is the rowing boat.

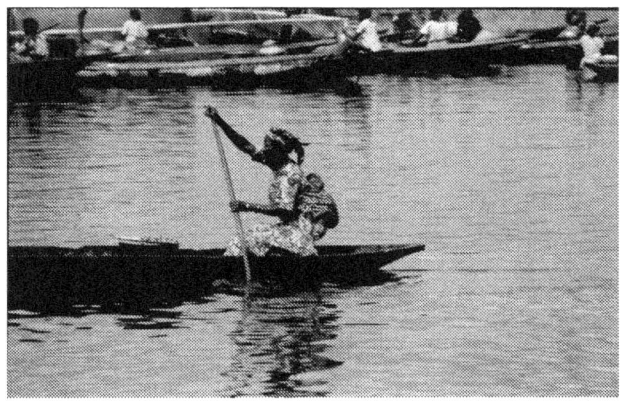

Picture 12: Ganvie village. Time has stood still here for centuries.

The men fish whilst the task of drying, smoking and selling the fish falls to the women. At the end of each day, smoke rises above the thatched roofs and the smell of fried fish spreads far over the lagoon.
In the morning, countless boats are loaded with dry fish, fruits of the surrounding area and other goods, gathered together on the village's colourful floating market.

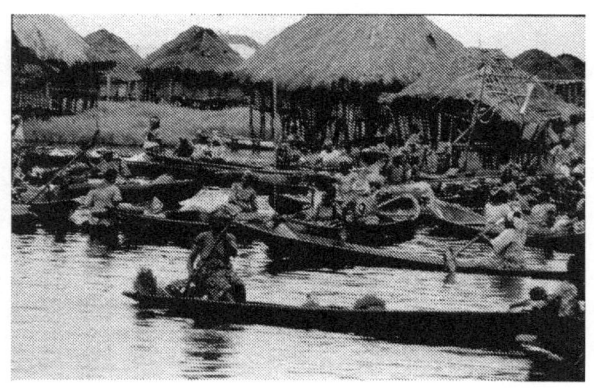

Picture 13: Ganvie village. The floating market.

The goal of our journey was the Penjari National Park in the north west of the country. We were warned that the road ahead, some 700km, was difficult to pass but we set out anyway. The paved road, starting from Cotonou, soon disappeared and passing through Savalou, we became involved in a local Christmas festivity.

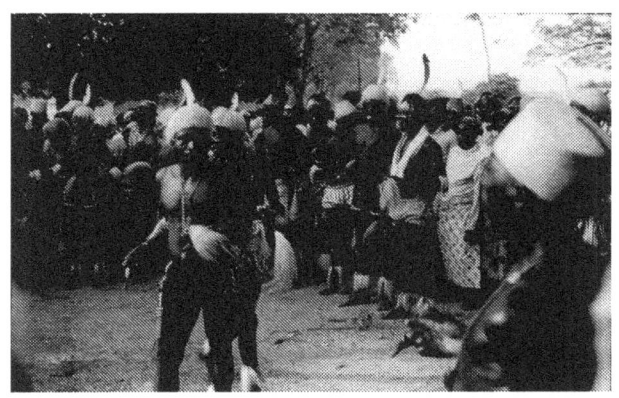

Picture 14: Djougou area – Middle Benin. The partly traditionally dressed natives danced happily.

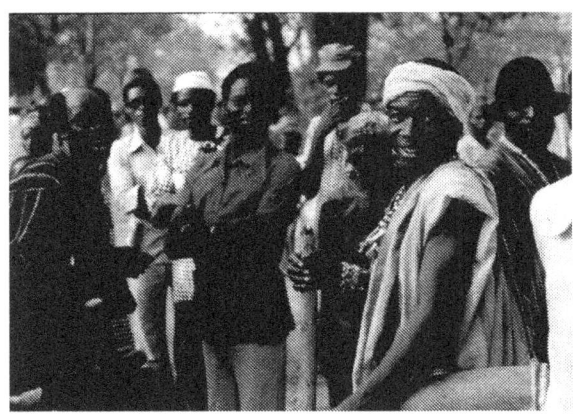

Picture 15: Djougou area. The joyful crowd.

The people had succumbed to the influence of palm wine and as we didn't speak their language, we continued on our journey.

After only a short time, the car's air-conditioning system broke down. It was not long before we were covered with dust from the open windows. Dust was something we had to get used to in Africa. It accompanied us on every step, during long trips, safaris or walking in the bush on dirt tracks. And with the dust came the heat.
A few hours later, well into the bush, we saw some strangely built red adobe
"castles". It was at this point we knew we had arrived at the Somba tribe's area.

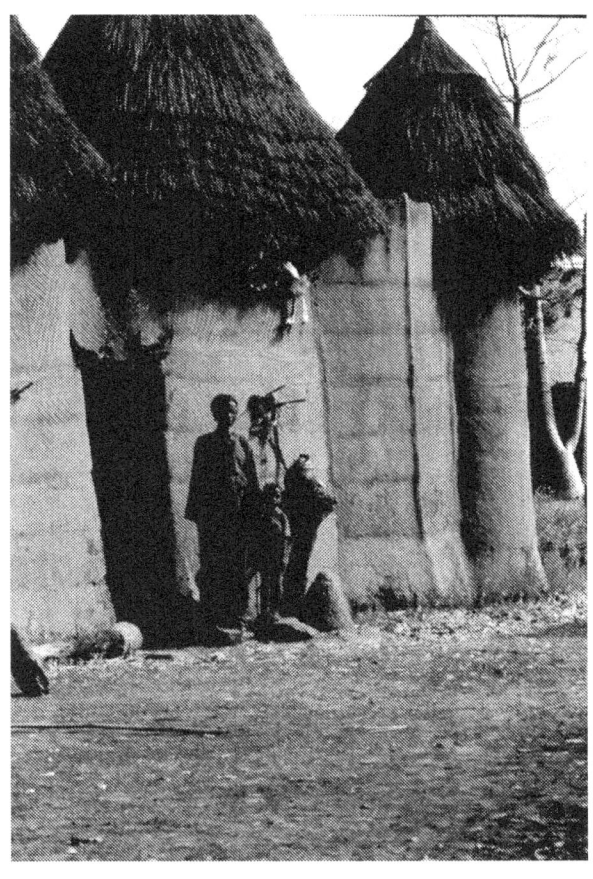

Picture 16: West – Benin. The "castle". Typical Somba building in the bush.

We got out of the car and approached a group of interesting-looking buildings. On closer inspection we saw that different animal parts were hanging on the walls of this strange-looking "castle". As we looked around, some stones were suddenly thrown at us from the bush. We soon hopped back in the car and with a roar and a large dust cloud, we drove away.

The Somba live in the western part of the country, hidden away deep in the bush. The men of the tribe are still hunters. Out of red clay, they construct spectacular - castle–like houses, without windows. The houses are usually built in the form of several round tower-like buildings, joined together.

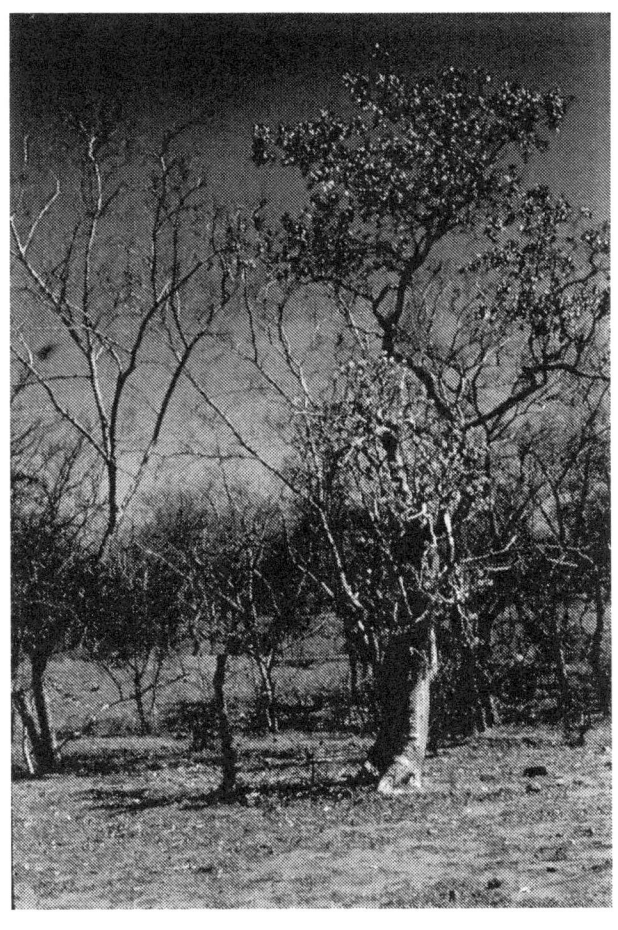

Picture 17 : Desert rose in the bush. Indigenous people make arrow poison from the white sap and seeds.

Near the Penjari National Park, we spent the night in a small hotel run by a French couple. Early the next morning, we headed to the park, eagerly awaiting our adventures, but during the course of the day, we encountered only a few hippos.

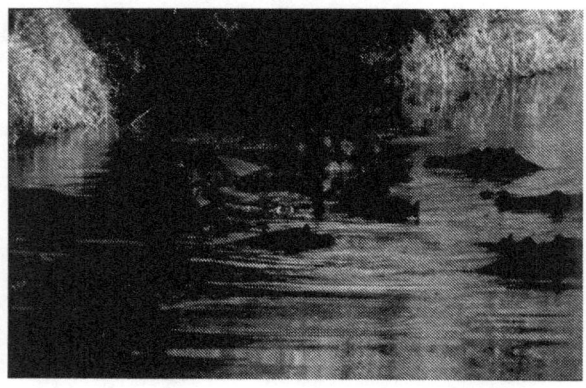

Picture   18:   Penjari National Park in Benin. Hippos.

The red disk of the sun touched the edge of the horizon. We had run out of water. The car slowly moved on the dirt paths, criss-crossed with wadis, then slipped and didn't want to start again. We fiddled with the engine, oblivious to the possibility of attack from wild animals, whilst many tiny flies came to take a closer look. It became more and more difficult to keep our eyes open. Night fell rapidly, all of a sudden, and it seemed as if we were going to have to sleep under the stars. But we were lucky, for a pair of headlights approached and an English driver towed our car to the nearest village. Whilst the car was being repaired, we slaked our thirst in the local "pub".

Next day, we aimed to return to Nigeria by the shortest route, as the last day of the year was looming and we wanted to spend it at home.

On the way, it started to rain hard. There was no trace of any inhabited area and the bush grazed the car as we tried to follow the wheel-marks etched in the mud in front of us. It was a nightmare. Just after midnight, we crossed the border into Nigeria at Kainji and found lodging in a roadside bush hotel. There was no other choice.

The room had no door, only a dirty cloth hanging on the door-frame. I knew it was pointless to dream about the Sheraton in Cotonou, where we had spent Christmas only a few days before. But finally, we arrived safely back in Kaduna in time for New Year's Eve.

The Voodoo Cult

In the 15th century, the Portuguese discovered the coasts of Africa . The European's interest increased as numerous expeditions were despatched to the unknown continent. These expeditions often did not succeed, as the unfriendly tribes dealt ruthlessly with the intruders. For this reason, the inner parts of the continent, even up until the mid-19th century, were all but unknown. During the same period, trade along the coasts flourished. For the white races, the alluring gold, ivory and slave markets produced large profits over the centuries. It also meant good business for the black slave traders too.

The voodoo faith was born in Benin [Dahomey]. In the midst of the slave trade era, the slaves and their faith reached South America and the Caribbean, where the gods of the Yoruba mixed with biblical figures. The voodoo cult arrived back on the south west coast of Africa during remigration, mostly to Ghana, Togo, Benin and the western parts of Nigeria. Even now, this faith is very much alive and well.

In the event of any misfortune, the head of the family performs a sacrifice to the spirits at the house altar. He puts food, oil, gin, and palm wine in front of the altar and then calls on the demons and spirits. If nothing happens, it means the gods are demanding a blood sacrifice.

Over the centuries, the rites and rituals of the different religious ceremonies were taken over from the Yoruba by the people living on the west coast.

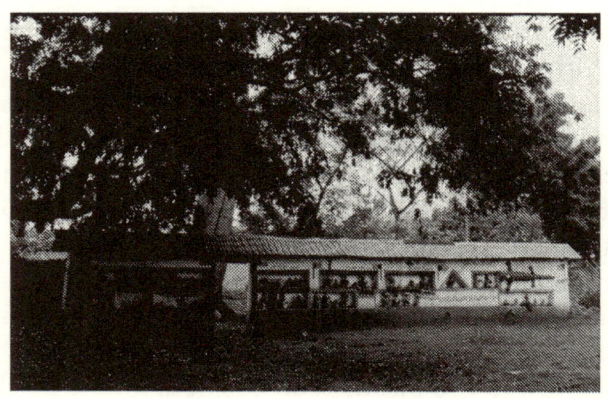

Picture   19: Near Cotonou – Benin. Fetishes.

The most important instruments of the voodoo cult are the idolised figures [fetish], which are charged with magic power. The mysterious bewitchings, beliefs, obscure deaths, resurrections from the dead, healing and ecstasies are all built on black and white magic.
The voodoo gods are frequently hostile, but may help people as well. Some of them are humane and will accept food or drink and tobacco, but mostly they demand blood sacrifices. This faith gives the followers a superstitious dread and its people are afraid of evil spirits, bewitching and the revenge of the dead.

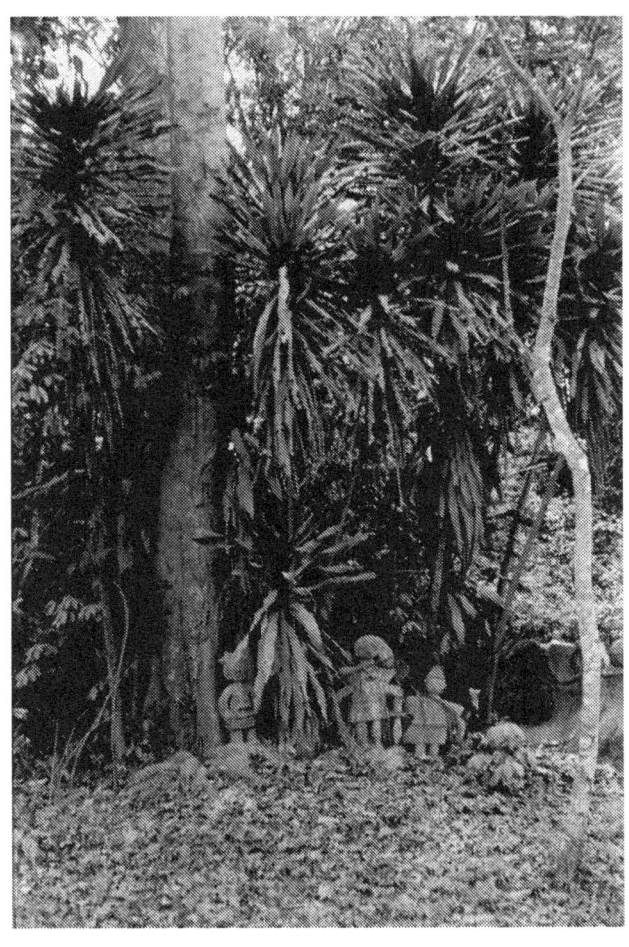

Picture 20: Voodoo dolls [fetishes] somewhere in the bush, near Cotonou, Benin.

Before ceremonies, the body or simply the face of the participants is painted white with kaolin.

At the beginning of the ceremony , the priest pours gin, whisky or any other spirit under the altar as a gift to the gods. He then sprays the rest of the drink in three different directions whilst murmuring prayers. In the meantime, drums are beaten in front of the temple, and a woman starts to dance, closely followed by others.

With this ritualistic dance, the women are asking the gods to remove evil spirits from their bodies. Although trance is a vital part of the ceremony, not everyone is able to reach this state. If the gods possess the dancing body, the rotation gathers speed and the dancer falls into a trance and therefore loses herself. It's very spectacular to watch and evokes excitement in the onlookers.

WEST AFRICA

NIGERIA

Nigeria is the most populated country in Africa with a population of approximately 120 million. There are about 250 different ethnic groups. The biggest are the Hausa, Kanuri, Nupe and Fulani, all of whom live in the north, the Yoruba and Edo in the south west and the Ibo in the south east. Although the official language is English, the different ethnic groups speak their own tribal languages.
The country has a tropical climate with alternating rainy and dry seasons. Precipitation is very low in the north but gradually builds up southwards.

Nigeria gained independence in 1960 following British colonial rule. From the '70s it became one of the world's largest crude oil producing countries and soon became rich and self-sufficient. Development started but revenue from oil production alone was not enough to meet the expectations of the fast growing population. Unskilled, uneducated masses have left the rural areas behind to try their luck in the cities and as a result, agricultural output has spiralled into recession, with exports of groundnuts coming almost to a complete stop.
The well developed and most populous cities of the country are Lagos, Ibadan and Kano.

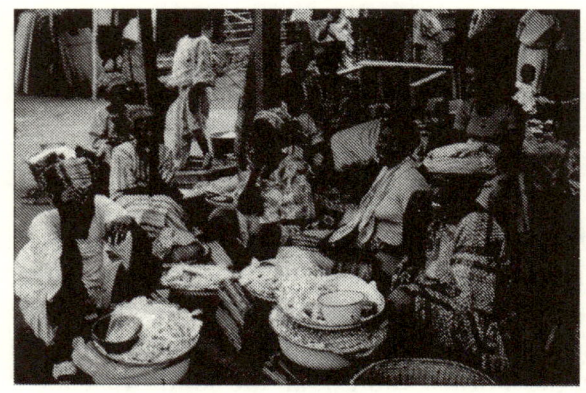

Picture 21: Ibadan. Yoruba market-women.

In Ibadan and Lagos, the Yoruba women organise themselves into well-run groups, thus ensuring their role as the heart of the business world.

The great metropolis of Lagos is busy day and night. The humidity is often around 90 percent. This wet, tropical heat is extremely difficult to cope with. The glistening modern city continues to expand to this day, outgrowing the slums which quickly reappear a bit further away. In the shade of tall tower blocks or under the great flyovers or in between alleyways, hundreds of thousands of people engage in a little bit of buying or selling, ever hopeful of a small profit. This chaos is increased by the throb of traffic on the multi-lane streets, which sometimes become paralysed for hours. Vendors swarm to the stationary cars and, underbidding each other, they offer an amazing variety of goods, just to earn a few [kobo] pennies.

The richest quarters of the city bustle with life. The beautiful villa-quarter with its lush gardens reflects the riches within. Day and night, these precious gems are surrounded by high walls and guards who protect the homes from burglars. Burglary is still a daily occurrence, however. We experienced this in our Kaduna home.

For a long time, we employed a Hausa night guard [magardi] who was extremely proud of his poisoned arrows. One night we were awakened by loud cries and after a few minutes, the magardi emerged from the green woods of the garden, announcing that he had finished off the burglars for good. He claimed to have shot one of them with his poisoned arrow and this burglar would therefore shortly die.

Did we believe him? Yes and no. But from that time onwards, there were no more break-in attempts.

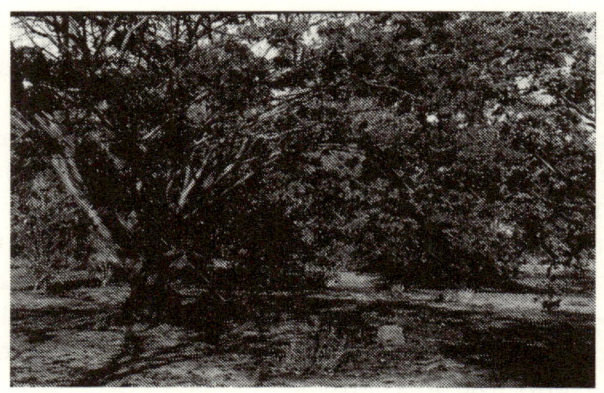

Picture 22: Our garden in Kaduna. Flame tree.
In bloom, scarlet flowers spread over the crown of the tree, forming what looks like a beautiful giant bouquet.

The countryside

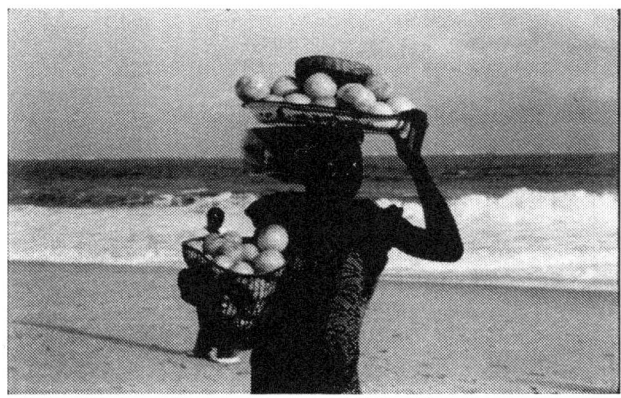

Picture   23:   Lagos. Yoruba fruit seller on the beach.

On the palm-fringed south west coast, the waves of the Atlantic continuously lash the beautiful untouched beaches.
The Yoruba live in the south west part of the rain forest, where most of them are engaged in agriculture. The main crops are tobacco, sugar cane, cotton, cocoa, coconut, palm oil, cassava [manioc], and many kinds of fruit, such as orange, lemon, grapefruit, banana paw-paw, mango and pineapple.
The women usually sell these exotic fruits in the market or along the roadside. Sometimes, roasted bush rats are also offered, stretched out on crossed sticks.

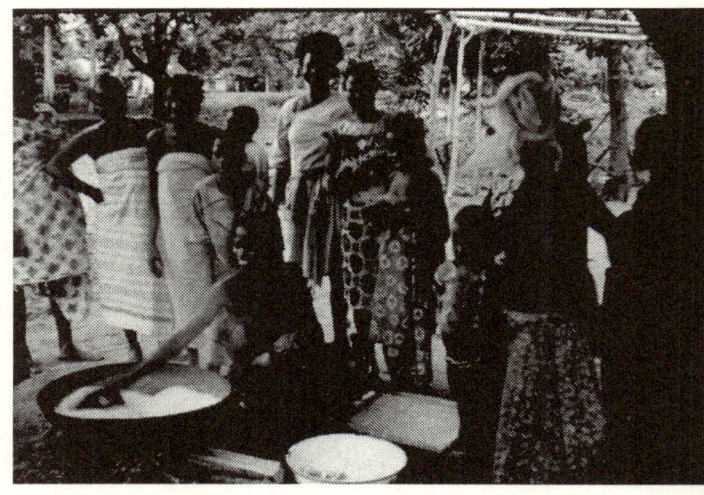

Picture 24: Yoruba women around Ibadan.

The ground cassava [manioc; like the yam tuber, but smaller] needs plenty of stirring over the fire in order to remove the poisonous material from the flour. When cooked this is a popular food.

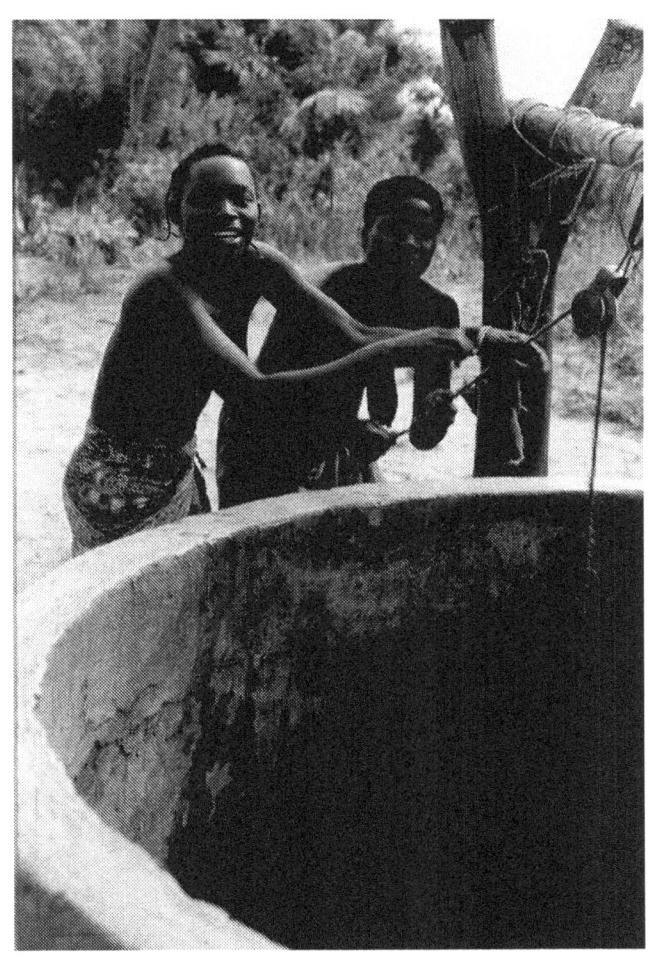

Picture 25: West of Nigeria. Around Ilaro. Yoruba girls drawing water from the well.

In smaller villages, the upper body of the women is usually naked, but below the waist they cover themselves with brightly coloured fabrics.

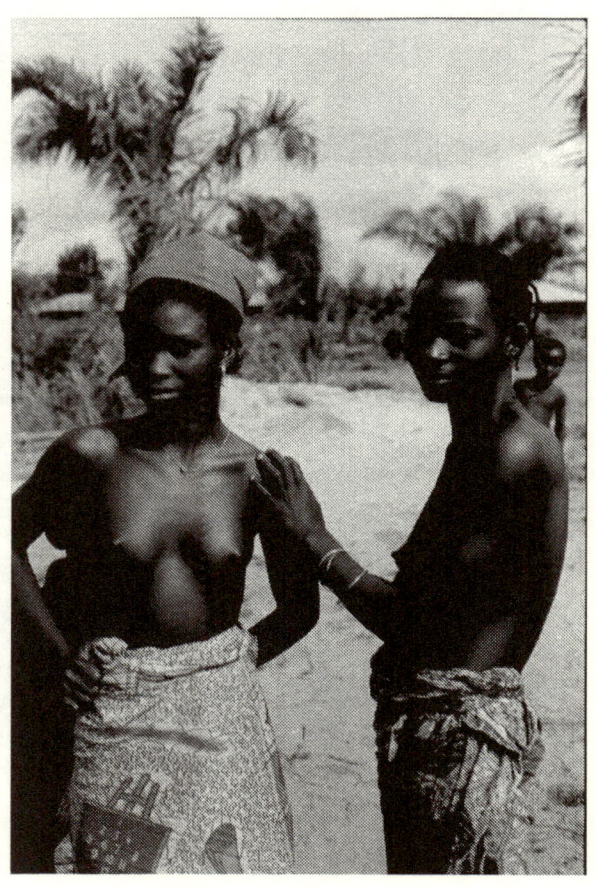

Picture 26: Around Ilaro. Concern.

From the bay of Benin [slave coast] onwards, about one third of the country is tropical rain forest. This dominant vegetation contributes to the health of the globe's ecological processes. Unfortunately, the local inhabitants are logging these great forests in order to gain more arable land. However, the thin topsoil quickly erodes as the rains wash off the humus layer, and the soil becomes infertile.

In the eastern part of the country, the landscape is very picturesque.

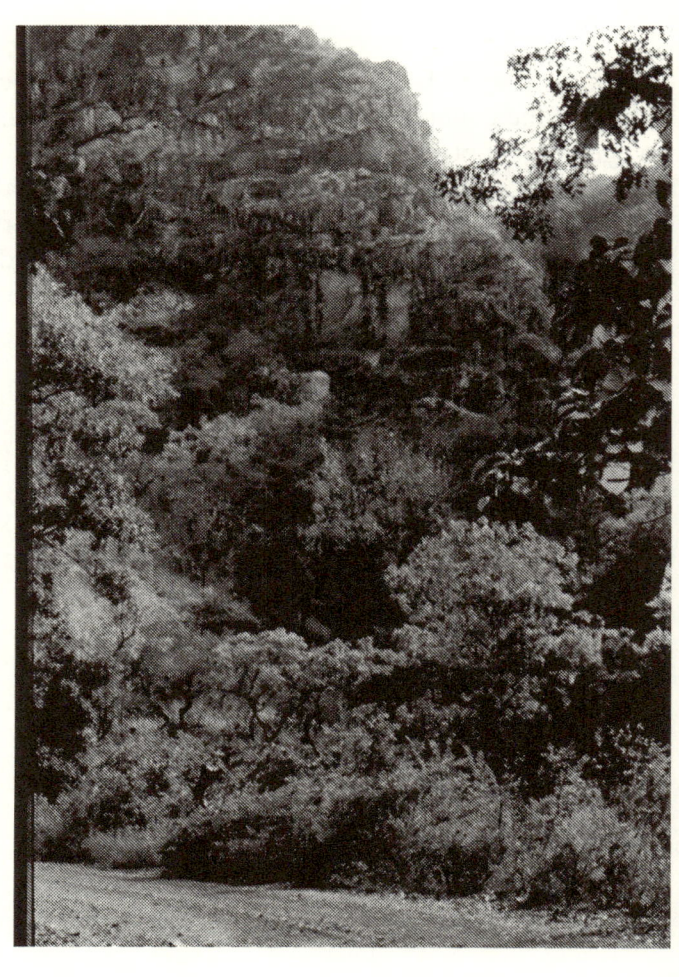

Picture 27: East – Nigeria. Close to the Cameroon border.

Located towards the north in the central part of the country is the plateau highland, which has its own particular terrain.

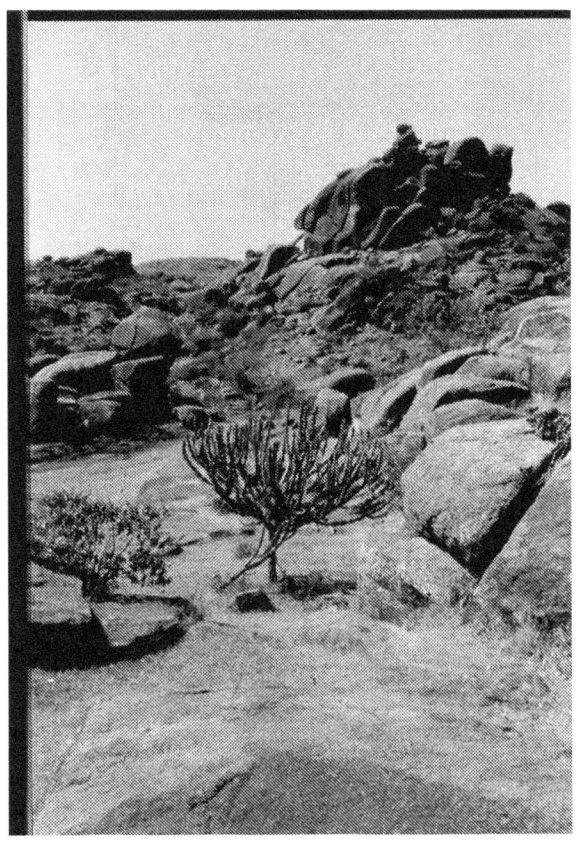

Pictures   28:   Jos. One of the strange hilltops.

Around Jos, hilltops reach skyward and in other parts, gigantic pebbles have been formed out of the granite outcrops as if a playful giant has put them on top of each other.

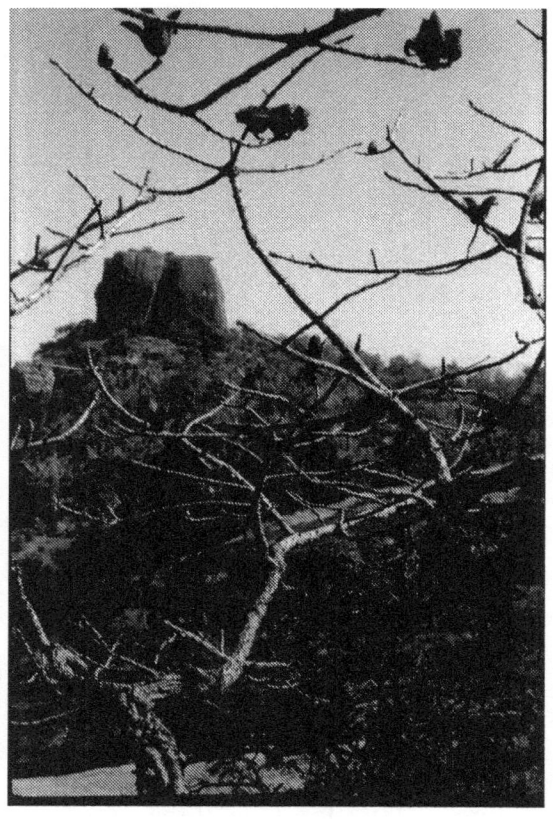

Picture 29: Jos. Beautiful landscape.

Here the countryside is fertile with good agriculture. During the rainy season, there are plenty of vegetables and fruit, including strawberries.

Not too far from Jos, the Yankari Game Reserve is well worth a visit. Baboons dominate and they scamper everywhere, stealing into the huts or the cars, and with lightning speed will snatch anything.
We once had an uninvited guest in our land-rover. The sizeable male didn't want to leave and after rummaging around, he was finally satisfied with a handful of bananas. There is also an excellent hot spring, which is very enjoyable.

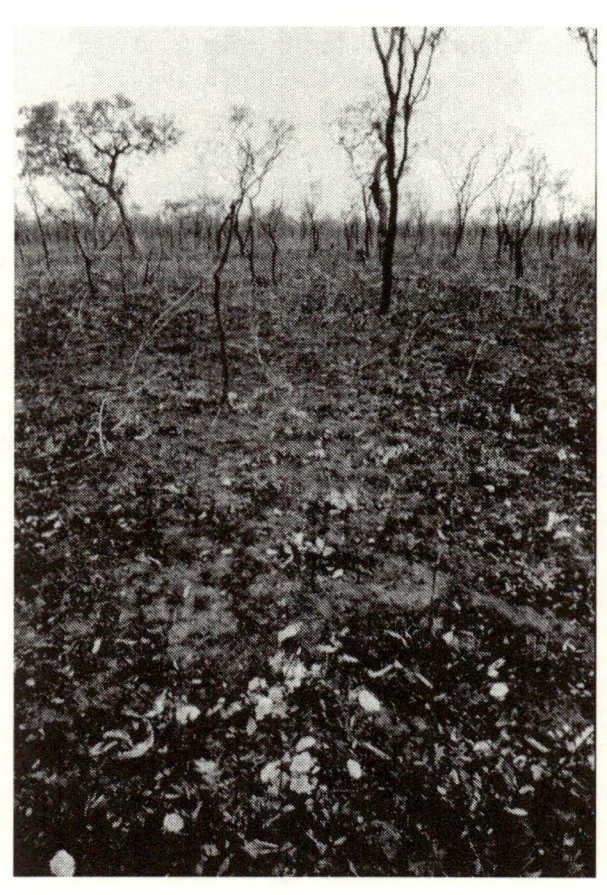

Picture 30: A part of Yankari Game Reserve burned down.

Following the destructive savannah fires, the territory of the wild animals temporarily becomes smaller.

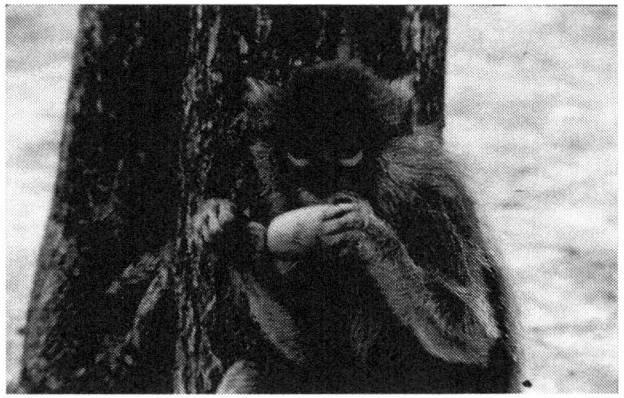

Picture 31: The red dancing monkey [Cerkof]. She was friendly and hungry.

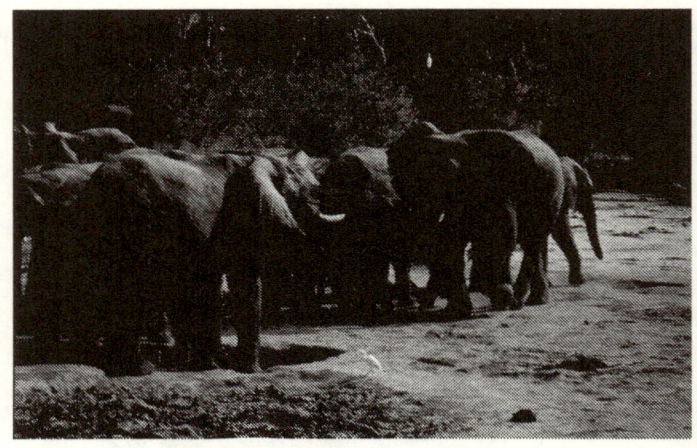

Picture 32: Yankari Game Reserve. Elephants at the salt pits.

With a bit of luck, you will sometimes spot elephants deep in the bush.

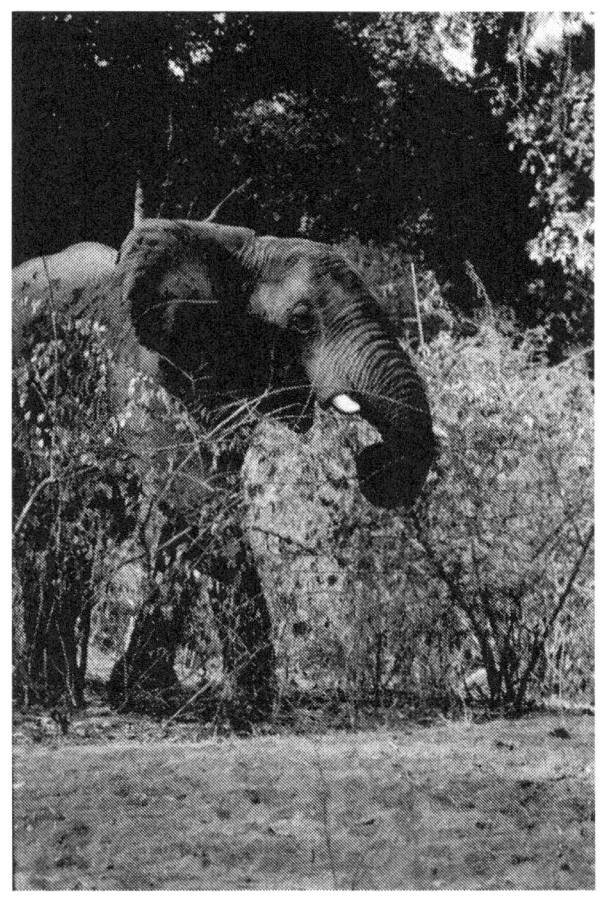

Picture 33: Yankari Game Reserve.

Walking in the bush, once, we suddenly noticed an elephant very close to us. It was alone, but after a few seconds slowly moved back into the bush. We were lucky, because it could easily have killed us.

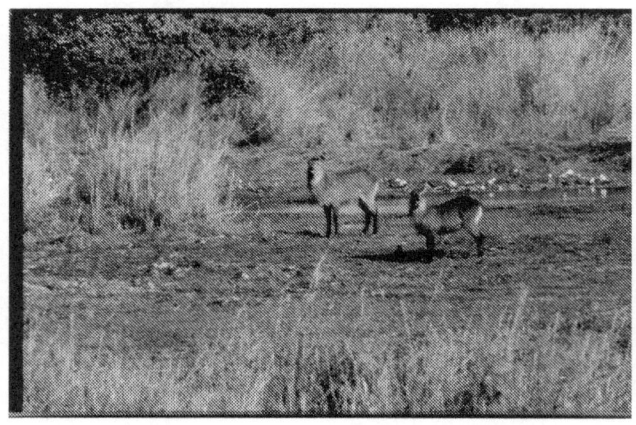

Picture 34:   Yankari Game Reserve.   Water buck.

Leaving behind the plateau highland, the woodland and bush savannah opens up and towards the north, the vegetation becomes more sparse. North east, however, in the flood area of Lake Chad, which may reach over 40kms across, dense bush covers everything.
On one of our several journeys, we wanted to see Lake Chad. We arrived at the village of Baga which is very close to the Lake. Unfortunately, that was the end of our journey as our car sank deep into the flood area. Some local men helped us to rescue the car but it was

impossible to continue our journey because of the mud. The shores of the water were still about ten kilometres away. So, disappointed we turned back.

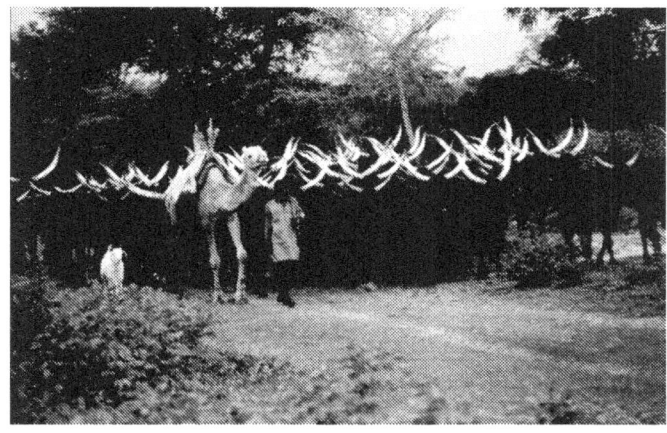

Picture 35: Bighorn cattle pass through the flood area of Lake Chad.

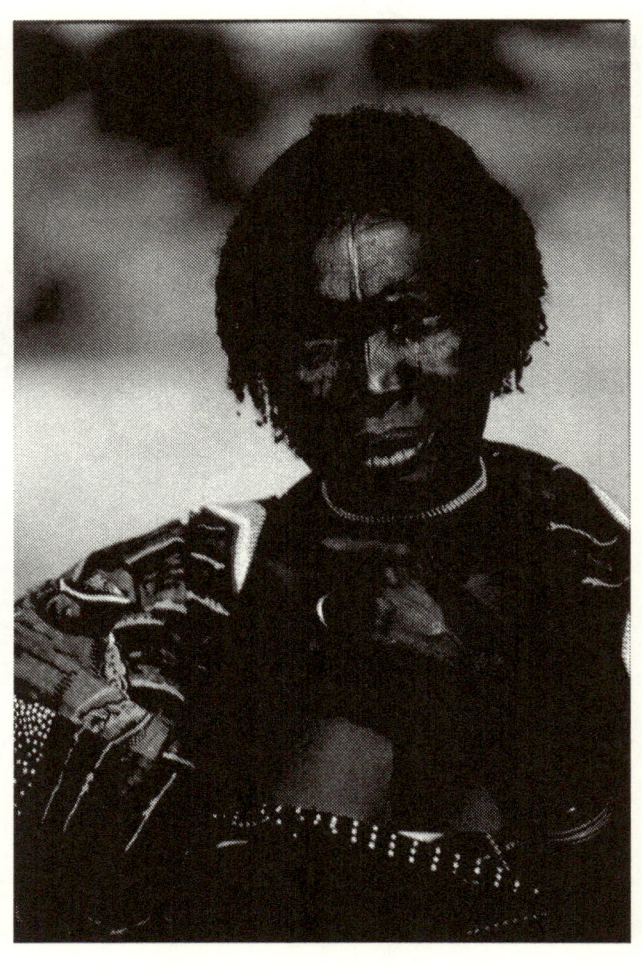

Picture 36: North East. Kanuri woman near the Chad border.

The Hausa, who follow the Islamic faith, live in the northern parts of the country. They are excellent traders, live in extended families, and polygamy is common. Their largest city is Kano and around this area are successful irrigated farms producing vegetables, chilli and even wheat.

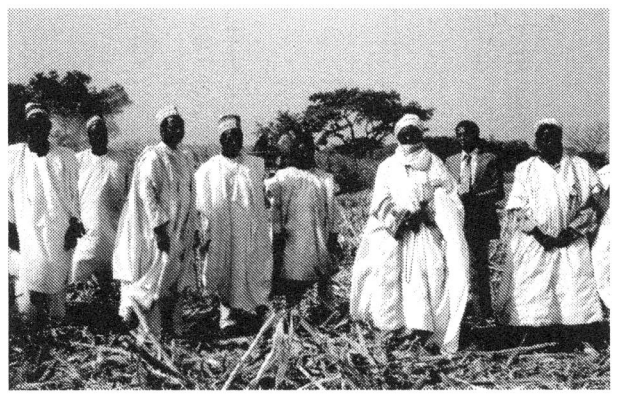

Picture   37: Hausa dignitaries inspect the maize harvest at the Kuzuntu demonstration farm. Their clothes [baba riga] were attractive, most of it richly embroidered.

Everyday life

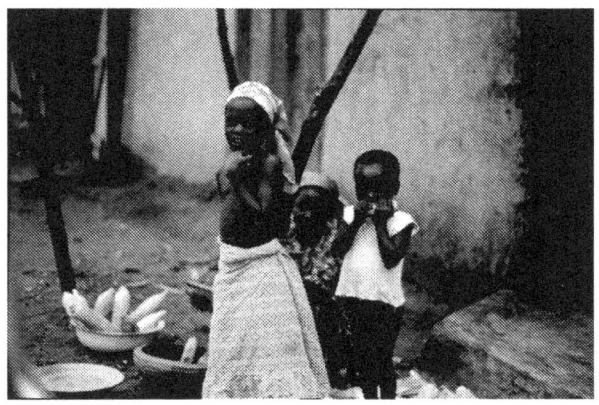

Picture 38: Kaduna. Young Hausa maize trader, with her children. In the earthenware pot, sweet smelling maize cobs are baked.

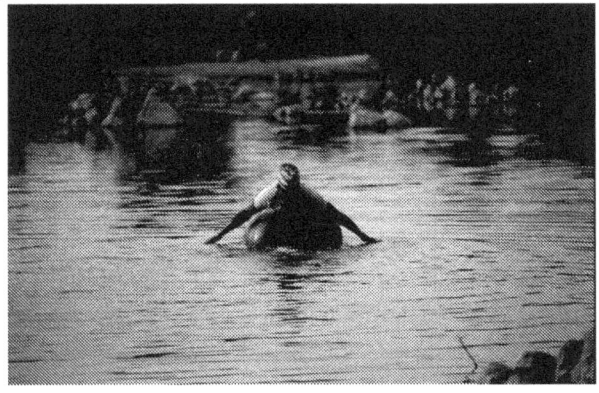

Picture 39: Kaduna. Hausa fisherman.

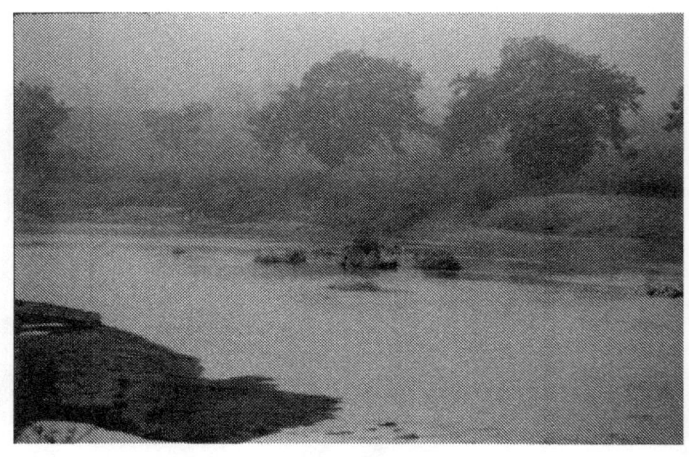

Picture   40: Harmattan over the river Kaduna. The hot dry wind carries dust from the desert.

From our home in Kaduna, we often travelled through the country, where poverty and malnutrition were a familiar and saddening sight.

In the villages, the unclothed, ragged children usually surrounded us with curiosity, extending their little hands as they asked for something.

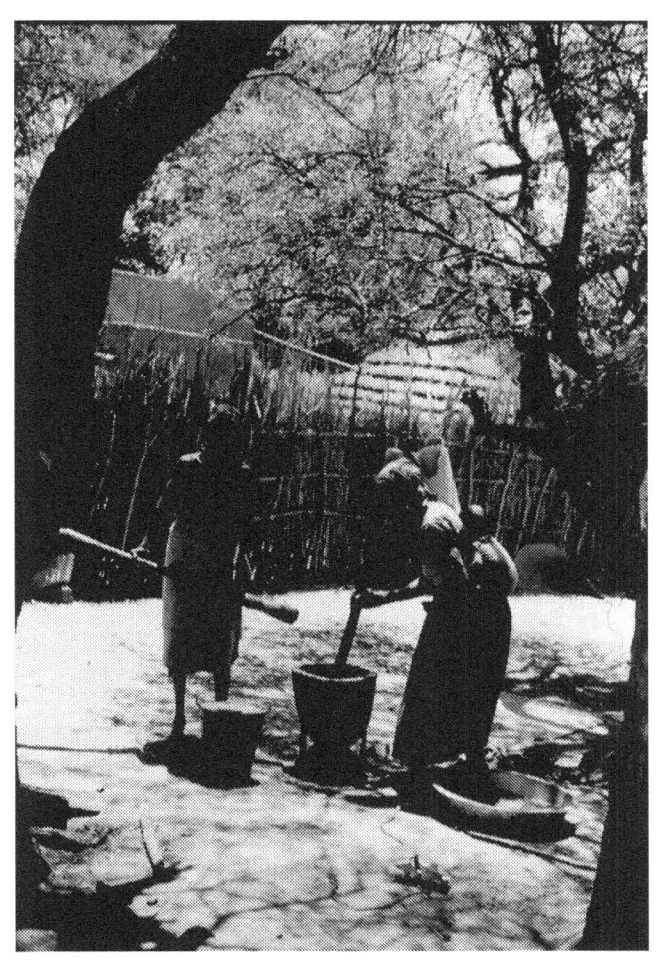

Picture 41: Near Kano.

Women crushing millet. In rural areas wooden mortars are commonly used. It is the duty of the women to crush the sorghum or millet for the preparation of flan or mash.

I can still hear the singing of the children through the window of a dilapidated school in Abugi.

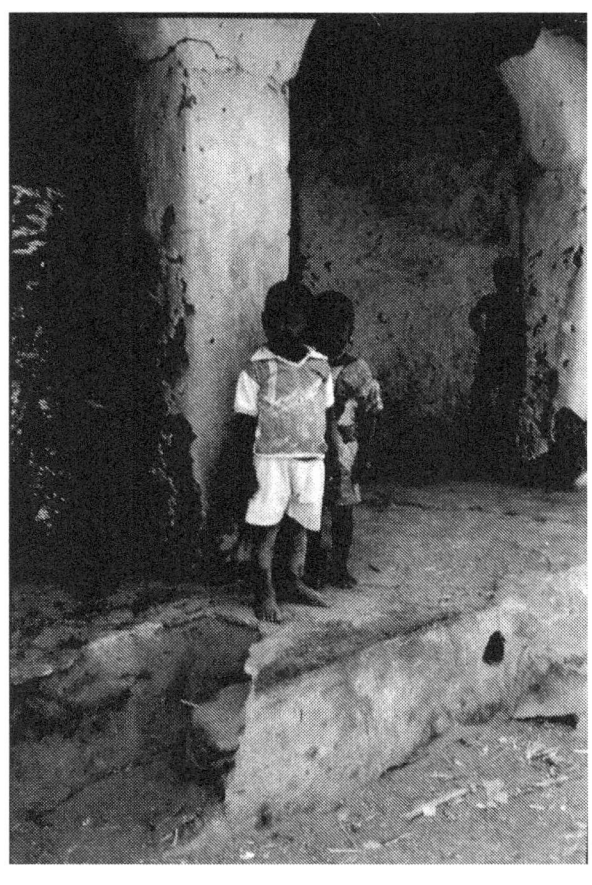

Picture 42: Abugi, Nigeria. In front of the school. These little children live in heart-breaking poverty. Most of them do not have any chance of quality schooling.

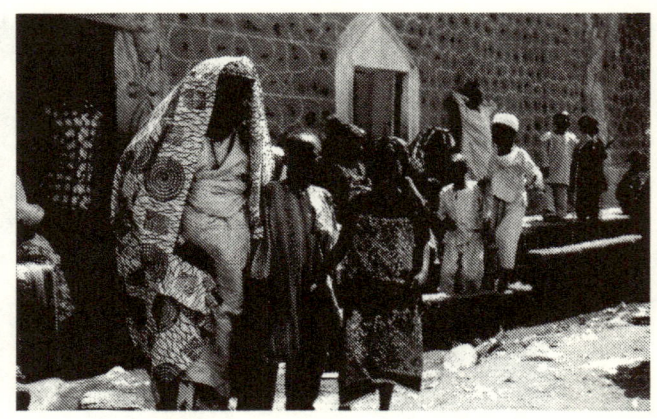

Picture 43: Zaria. Hausa grandmother with her grandchildren.

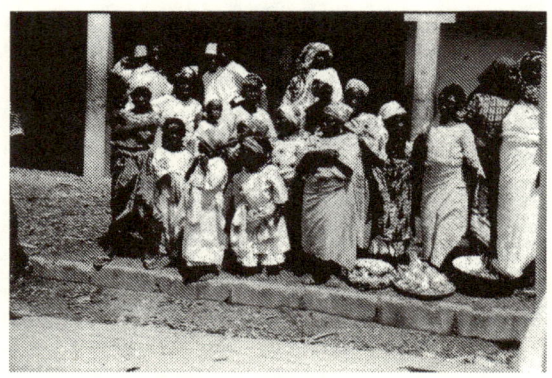

Picture 44: Zaira. Beautiful Hausa children in their best clothes.

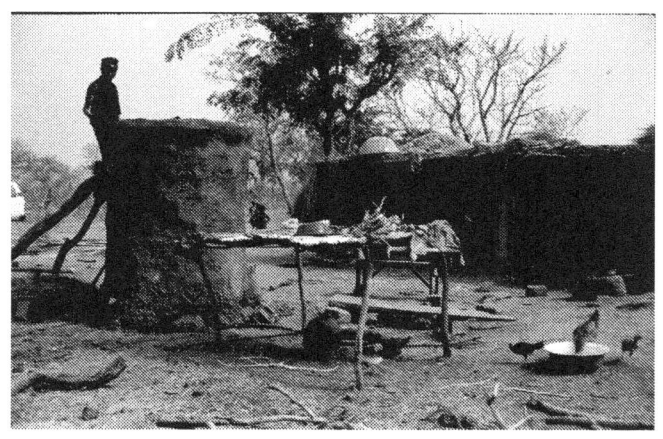

Picture 45: Kano area. Miserable hamlet. The man was building a granary, using only adobe. ''I hope, probably it will be full after harvest, if there is enough rain'' he said.

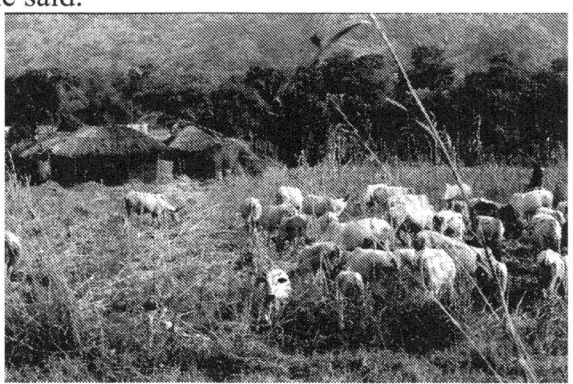

Picture 46: Bauchi area. Villages are often well hidden in the bush.

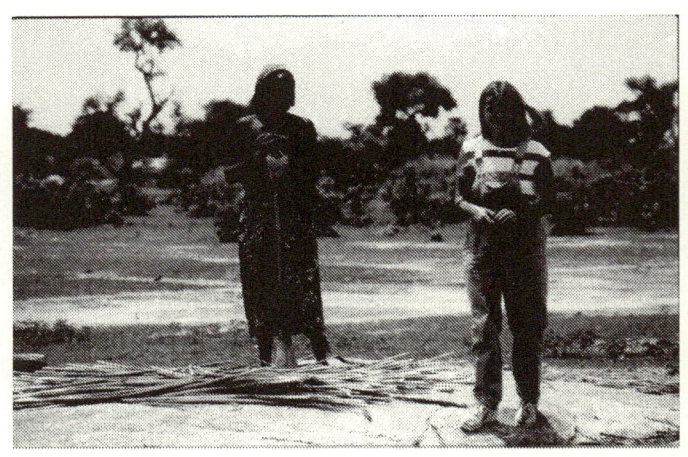

Picture 47: Around Abuja. Friendly Hausa woman threshing millet [and the author].

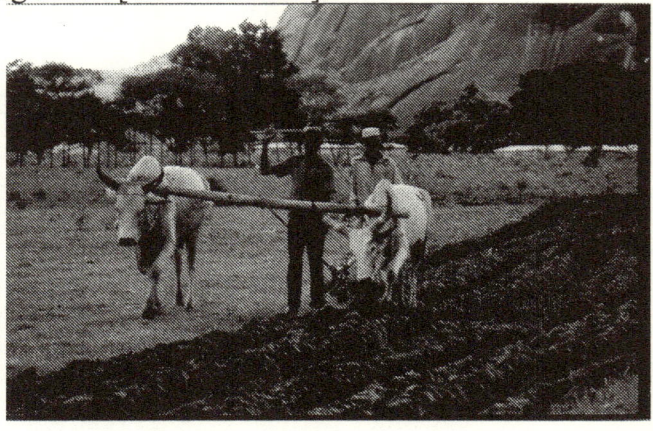

Picture 48: [Enlarge] Near Abuja. Around the smaller-larger settlements, people try to farm the land. Mostly they produce yam, maize, millet, cotton, groundnuts.

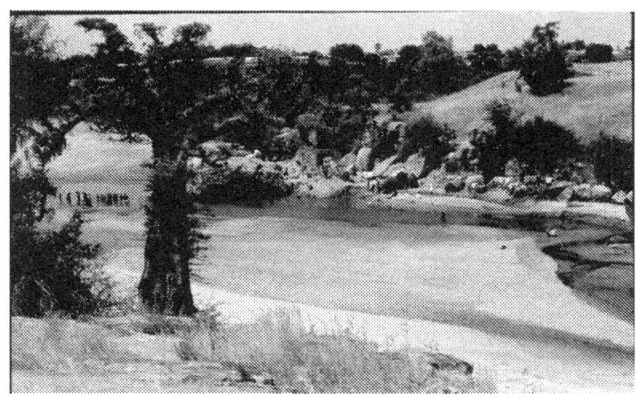

Picture 49: River Gongola in the dry season.
There is scarcely any water in the river bed once the dry season arrives. Locals use every last drop. They bathe, clean themselves and wash. Afterwards, they hang their clothes on the rocks or bushes to dry.

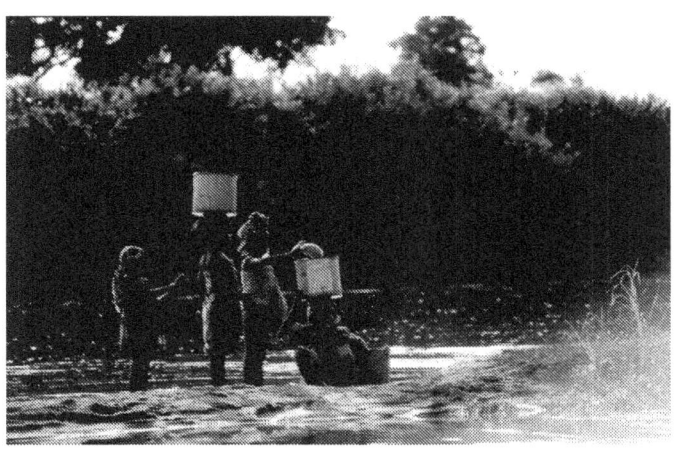

Picture   50: Central Nigeria. Abugi. Carrying water home from the river is an everyday duty, in which even the little girls must participate.

Deep in the bush

As we walked in the savannah, we often met the native people.
Far from the cities in the countryside, communicating with people was often impossible, as we didn't understand their language.

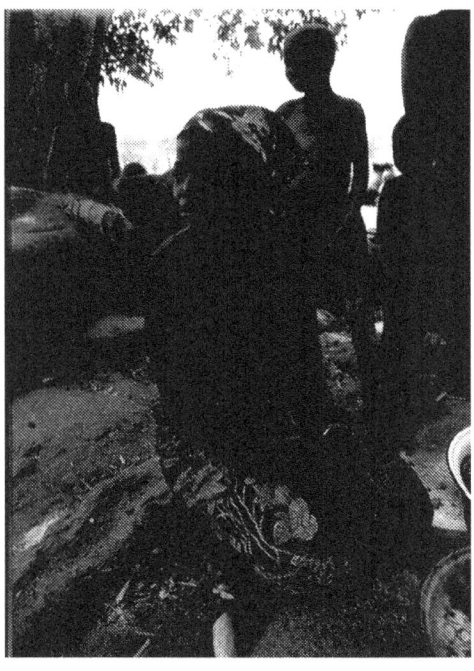

Picture   51:   Bauchi area. Zull village. The poverty. In the background, underfed children are gawking.

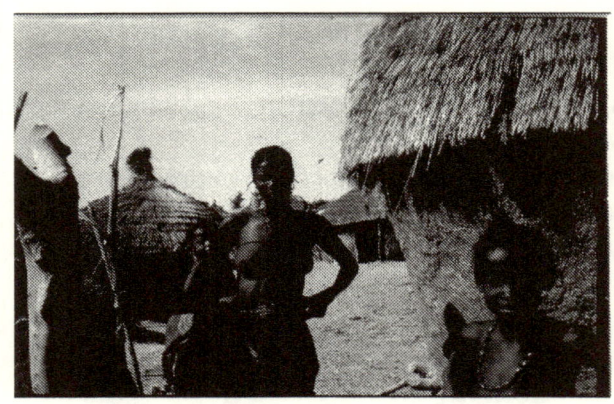

Picture   52:   North western area. Motionless, they watched as we approached. However their demeanour changed when we shook their hands.

The round huts are characteristic of the bush areas. From time to time, they repair the roof, which is made from millet stalks or long grasses. The walls are adobe, made by hand by the women.
They are built in a round shape due to the belief that evil lives in corners.
The women generally cook in front of the huts on an open fire. Once, we watched with surprise as on top of a blazing fire, a huge earthenware tub with suspicious looking liquid slowly bubbled. Pointing skyward from it was a hoofed leg.
There was no invitation to lunch.

The greater part of the northern region is still untouched savannah, home to the smaller nomadic groups. Their movement is determined by the weather, vegetation, water, and the need to avoid the tse-tse fly, which is the carrier of sleeping sickness.

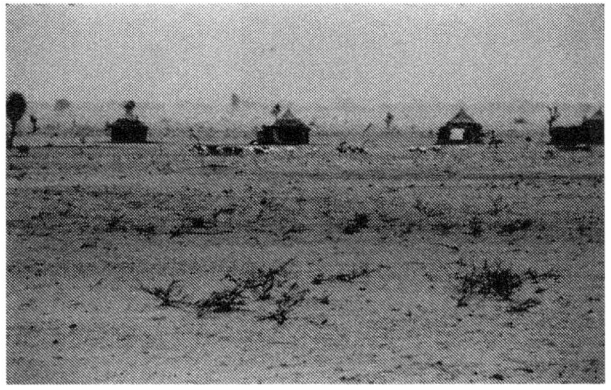

Picture 53: [Enlarge] North - Nigeria. The Wurno area is near to the southern part of the Sahara. Temporary settlement of the nomadic herdsmen.

Families live in simple huts built from millet stalks. Once, they allowed me to enter a hut. The inside was clean but furnished with only the grass matted bed and some household utensils.

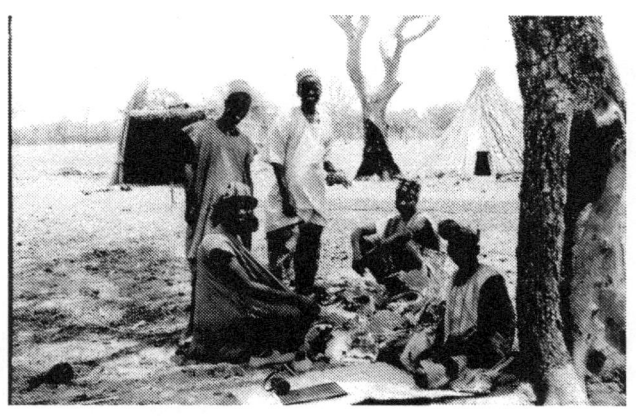

Picture   54: Near Kano. Hausa and Fulani men going about their business. This is the best way to buy fresh meat.

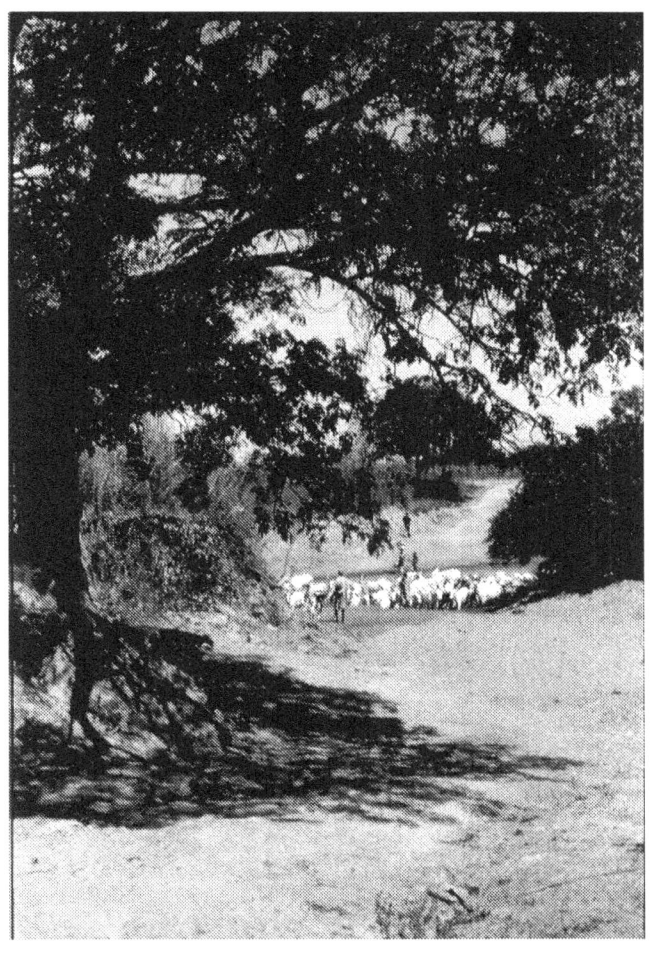

Picture 55: North - Nigeria. A nomadic herd crossing River Kuzuntu.

On meeting with a migrating Fulani family, a strange feeling settled in my heart, because I felt they lived in another world and the wonderful areas of the savannah belong to them. They do not care for civilised life. For generations, they have lived freely and they voluntarily stay in their own world, in spite of the modern rush and development.

It is easy to identify the Fulani as their faces are of a fine structure and their skin is not as dark. Some of the Fulani have settled but the majority of them are still scattered throughout the savannah.

I always remember coming across a small group gathering their belongings together as they prepared to leave. An old man with friendly clear eyes came over to us.

He greeted us and then stayed motionless for a while before waving his hand and following the rest of his herd.

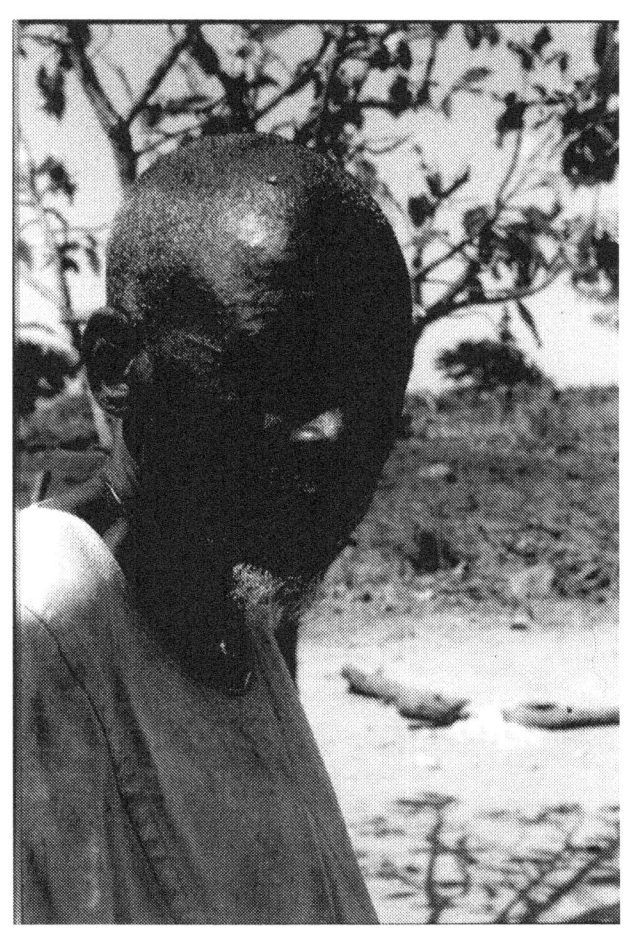

Picture   56:   Kano area. Fulani man.

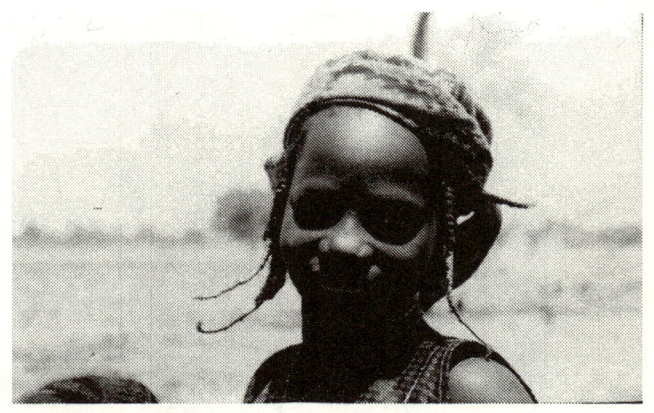

Picture 57: Little Fulani girl, somewhere in the savannah.

Markets
In the northern markets, the Tuareg are also present alongside the Fulani and other smaller tribes. These people draw attention to themselves with their different but interesting clothing, trinkets and beautifully hand-wrought weapons.

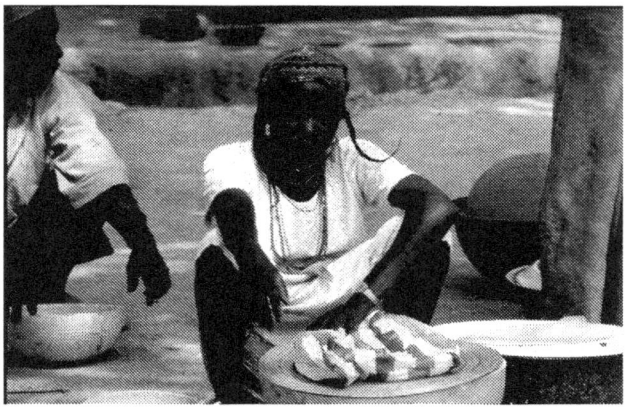

Picture 58: Kano area. In the local market a young girl waits for a customer.

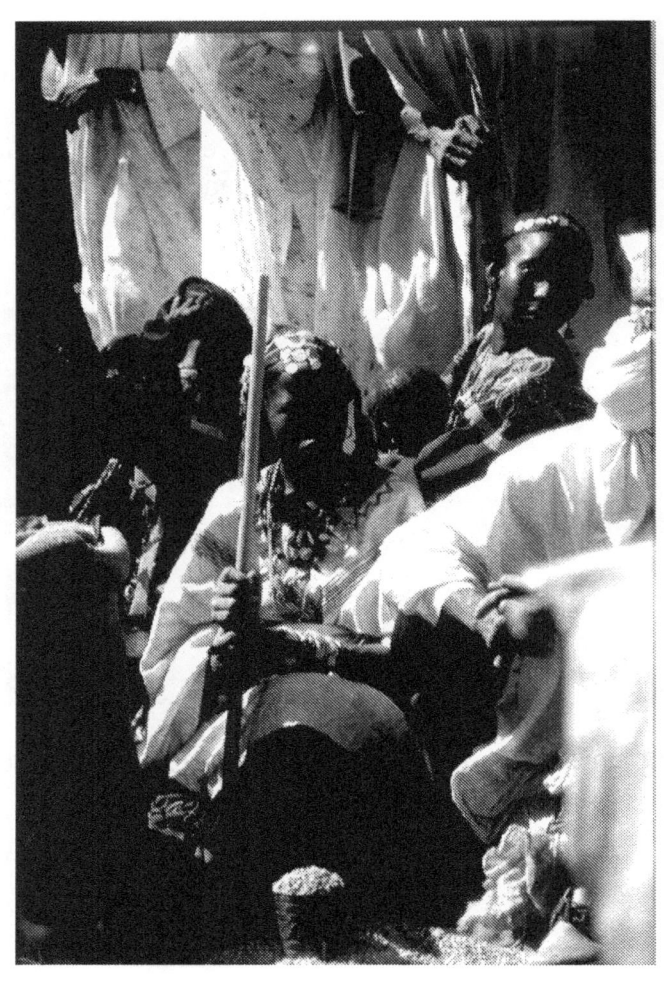

Picture 59: North of Kano. A beautiful Fulani women on the market.

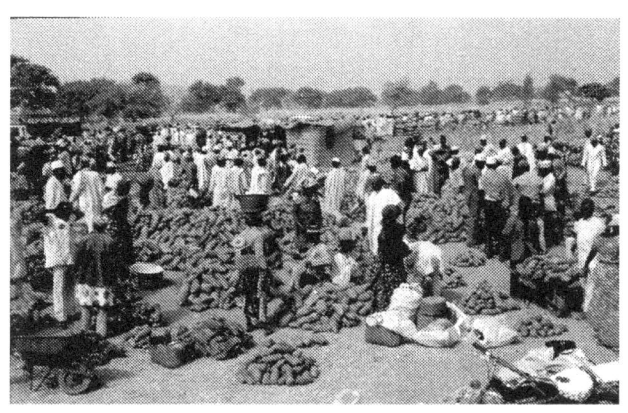

Picture   60: Near Kuzuntu. After harvest, special yam markets are usually held. The large tubers weigh several kilos. Yam is the staple food of Nigerians and when cooked, tastes a bit like potatoes.

In the markets of most villages, the locals buy and sell farm produce, vegetables and fruits. The butcher offers cut lumps of meat from his shaky table, whilst trying to keep the flies away. Beside him on the round barbecue, fragrant meat begins to brown, thick with the aroma of chilli. Anyone not accustomed to sharp spices would soon be sneezing.

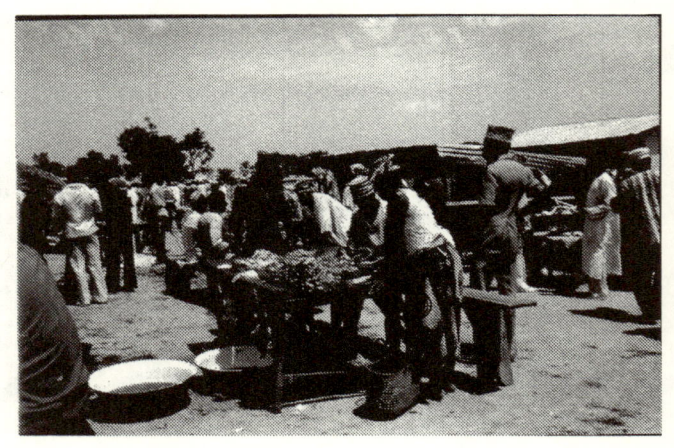

Picture 61: Kuzuntu. The butcher.

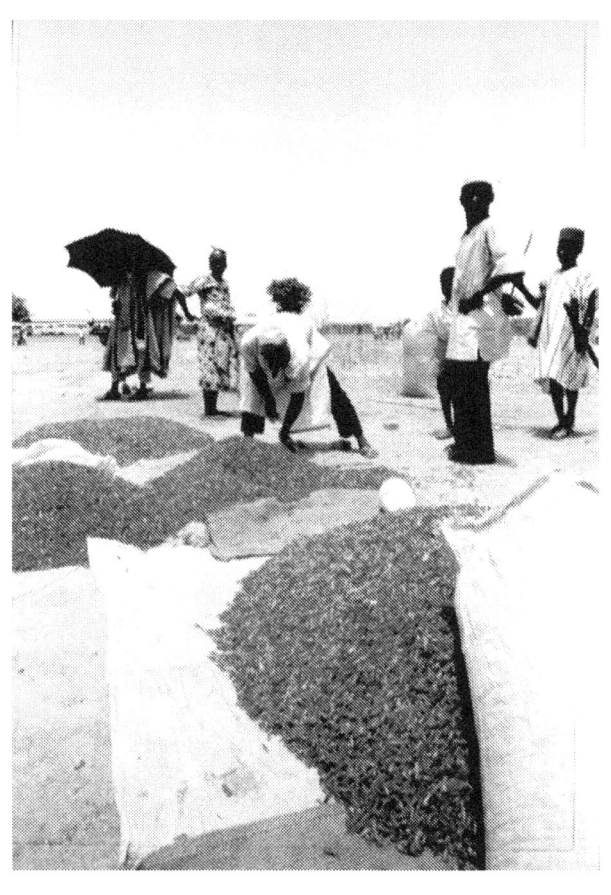

Picture 62: Kontagora. Chilli is a popular spice all over Nigeria.

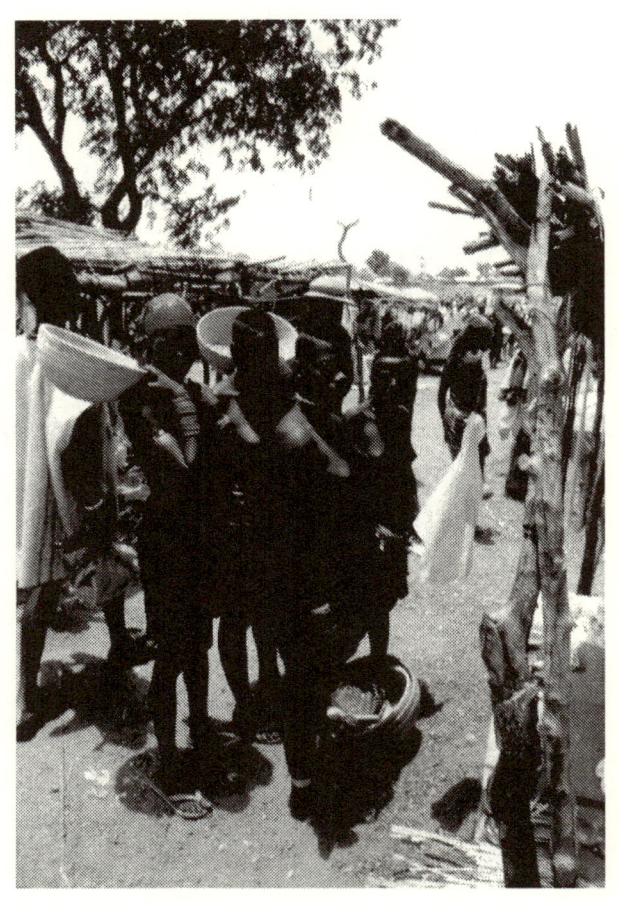

Picture 63: North West Nigeria. Suspicious Kambari girls. I wanted to speak with them, but they weren't very friendly.

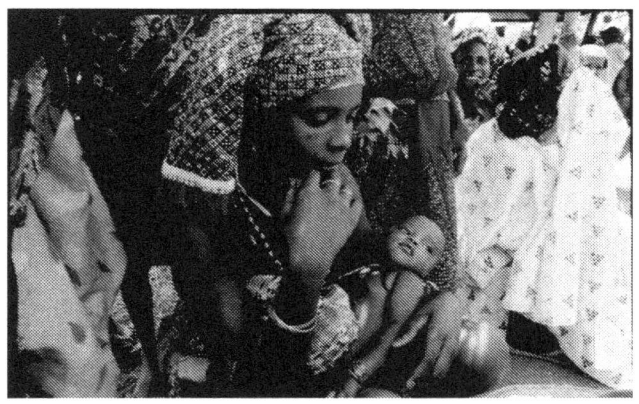

Picture 64 : West of Nigeria. Very young mother with her child. She was rather shy.

Culture & Folk art
The oldest archaeological discoveries in West African art have been found in the areas of Katsina, Ife, Abuja and Jos Plateau in Nigeria. The mystical terracotta heads and statuettes of the Nok culture date back about two thousand years according to estimates. The bronze heads and statuettes from the 9th Century are also of great value. It seems that a rather advanced level of culture may have existed in this region.
Over past centuries, due to the lack of written records, people have kept the events of history alive by oral tradition, with tales and songs. Beliefs and legends are superstitiously guarded and practised. Through war or trade, the tribes learned and exchanged ideas and customs and as a result, the practice of wood carving,

batik work, weaving, tanning and dyeing is still widespread.

The different ethnic groups [e.g.Yoruba, Edo, Ibo] used various materials such as iron, ebony, copper, bronze and ivory to produce astonishing masterpieces. To this day, people are still using these objects in ceremonies such as dances, birth, death, puberty, initiation, harvest or rain making.

The Hausa, Kanuri and Fulani groups living in the north are skilled in weaving, blue dyeing and tanning. Indigo dyeing is a tradition which goes back centuries in Kano and is still alive. Before dyeing, they design the pattern and tie small pebbles into the material. After dyeing, the spaces where the pebbles were remain lighter.

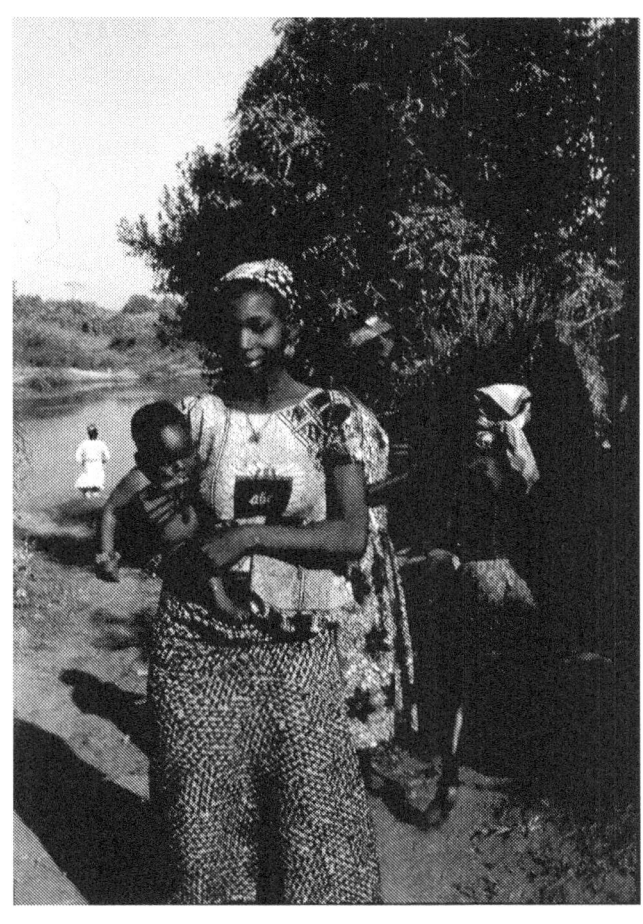

Picture 65: Kaduna. This Hausa woman is wearing a pretty patterned material around her waist.

In the old quarter of Zaria, one can find strangely built houses, where the facade is richly decorated with interesting geometric patterns and pinnacles. In the past, this Hausa town was surrounded by great walls built from sun-dried bricks. These and the gates are still visible.

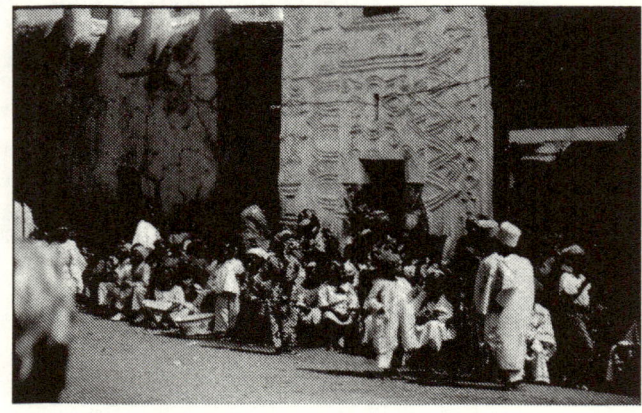

Picture   66: The oldest part of Zaria.

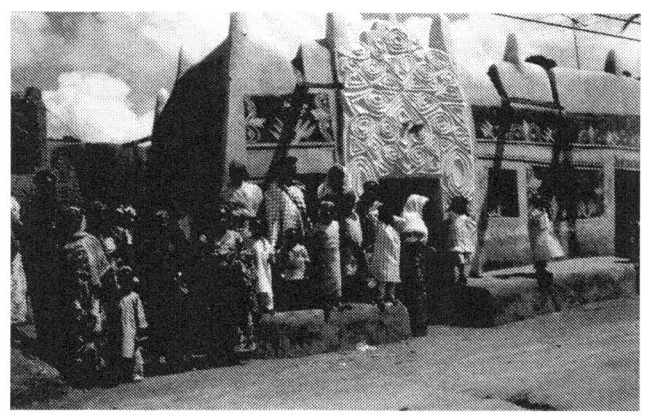

Picture 67: Zaria. Most of the old houses are richly decorated.

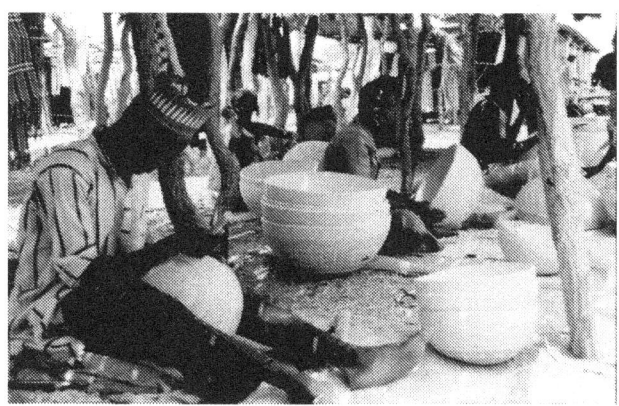

Picture 68: North West. A skilful Hausa artisan immersed in his work as he decorates the surface of a calabash with attractive animal images. The calabash

[gigantic pumpkin] is popular throughout Nigeria and is used as a storage vessel.

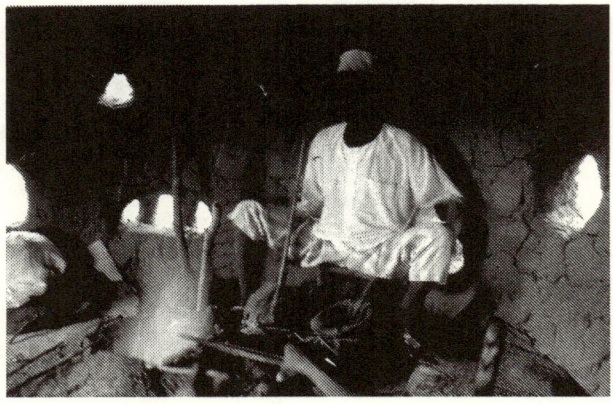

Picture 69: Nupe man. Glass beads are made in similar little workshops in Bida.
When we entered this little hut, the craftsman immediately made me a pretty bracelet – from a coca cola bottle.

The art centre of western Nigeria is Oshogbo, in the Yoruba area, where many artists choose to live. Their work, including gigantic statues, wood carvings and batik, is internationally recognised.

Body adornment, Scar tattoo, Dance
With the use of natural materials, such as seeds, stones, bones, grasses, leather, pebbles and shells, nomadic women are able to produce extremely attractive jewellery.

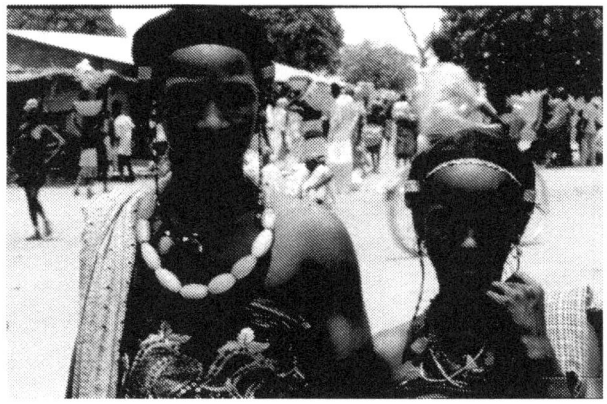

Picture 70: North West. These girls were very attractive.

People consider body adornment very important and their heads, necks, ears, and arms are heavily decorated with necklaces, rings, bracelets, amulets and even old coins.

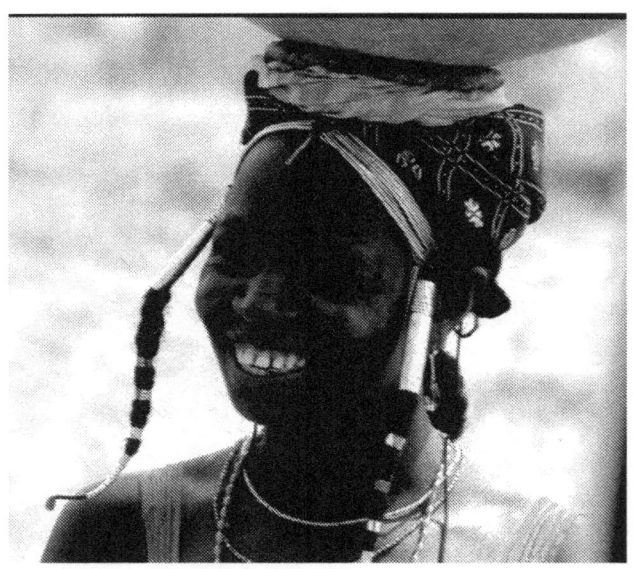

Picture 71: North – Nigeria. Often, gold wire is used to decorate the hair.

Women will draw attention to themselves with their elaborate jewellery, made of gold, silver or brass. Their faces are frequently painted with different signs and patterns.

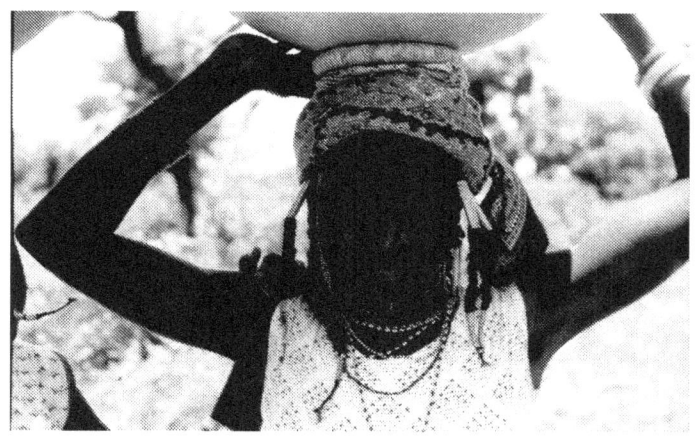

Picture 72: The young girls are also well decorated.

Even today in many parts of Africa, the cult of the body is very popular. Both sexes love body painting or intricate scar tattoos.

In rural areas, the upper part of the body is often naked and often densely covered with scar tattoos. These are made to a well thought-out pattern, with a series of tiny cuts. However, the process is painful and often carries a high risk of infection.

The tattoo is a ritual symbol, protecting the body from evil, and at the same time is highly decorative. Scars on the face are a mark of tribal identity.

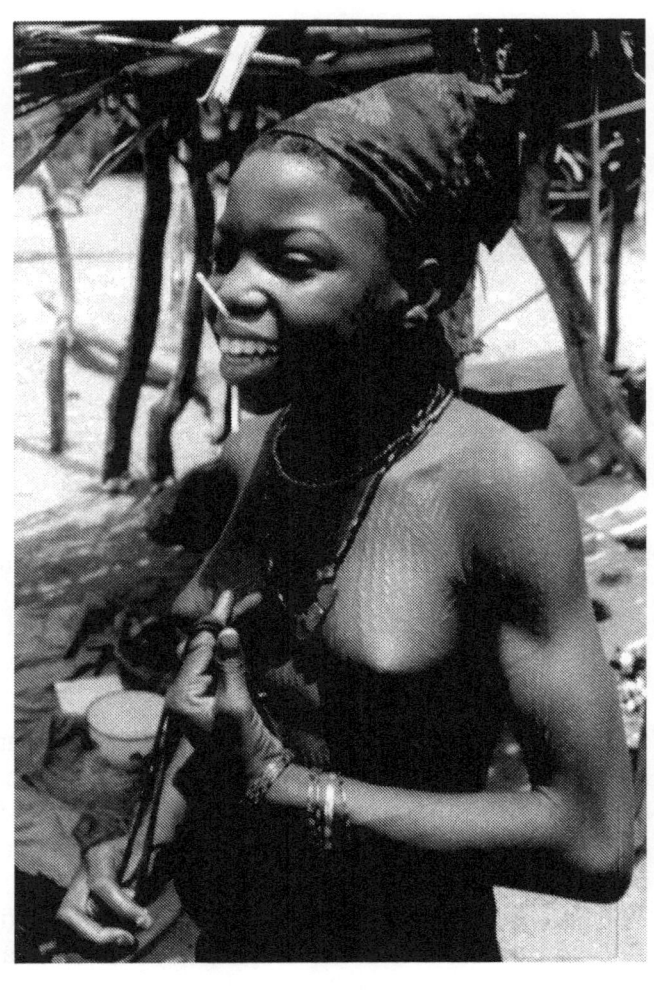

Picture 73: North West. Yang Kambari girl. Her body was intricately tattooed.

Africa would not be the same without dance and the sound of drums.
The movement of the people is both spectacular and expressive. The dance usually starts with slow marching steps but as the sound of the drums picks up speed, the body moves more and more quickly and expressively. The elderly also love to dance.

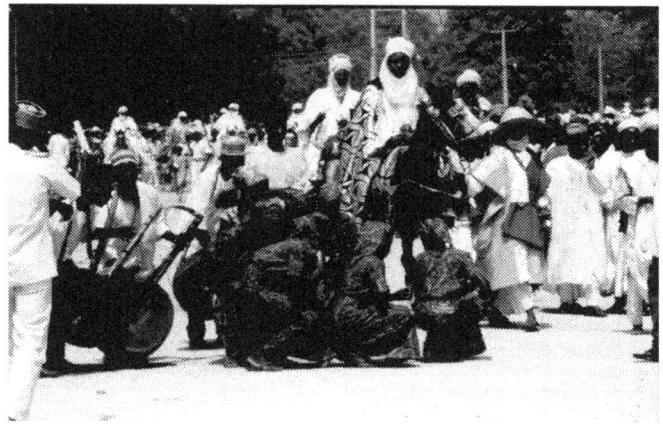

Picture 74: Zaria. Hausa women greet the arrival of high-ranking dignitaries with dance.

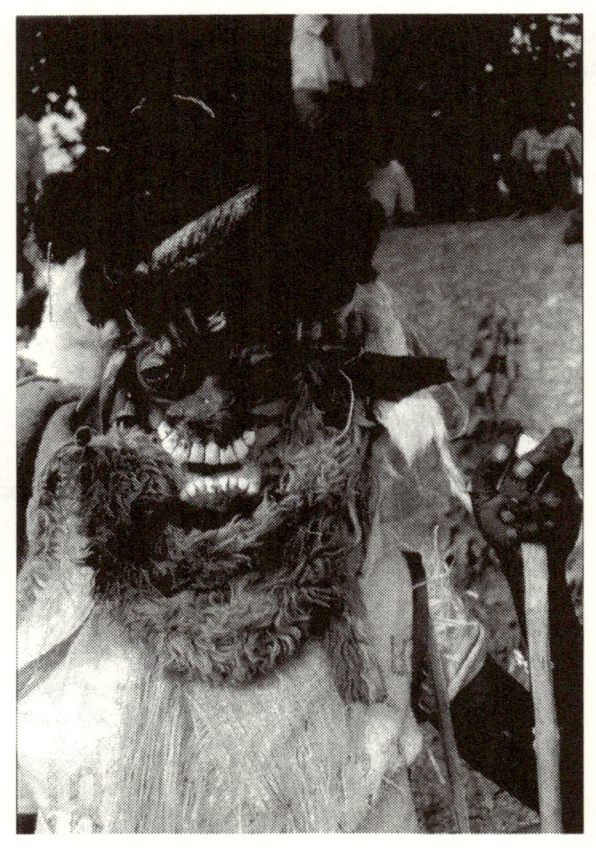

Picture 75: The Jos way. Fearsome mask.

Each ethnic group has its own festivities, where the most important elements are drums and masks. The Ibos are renowned for their mask making, a basic component to any spiritual festival. Such masks heighten the atmosphere and during the actual dance, help to create both frightening and magical impressions.

At night, over the blazing fire, the mask-wearing men elicit fear in their spectators with their magical dance. Far away from the cities, life changes, and around the evening fire, singing and drumming entices the crowd into a whirling, spiralling, thrilling dance. As the feet fly, the dust rises and showers a mystical layer over the red light of the fire.

Sallah Festival

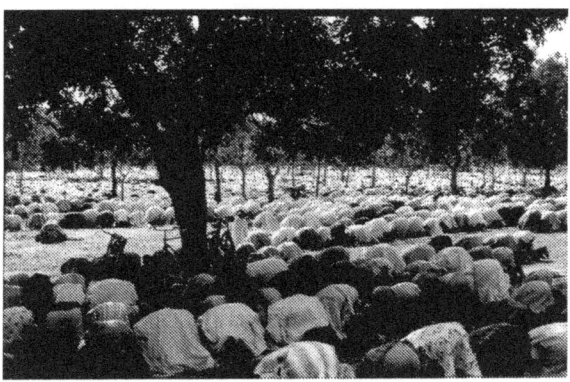

Picture 76: Zaria. The prayers.

In the Muslim Hausa territories, the most well known ceremony is the Sallah Festival. After forty days of fasting during Ramadan, hundreds of thousands of Mohammedans say their prayers. Afterwards, they hurry to the festival site, where everyone is waiting for the Emir and his lustrous escort.

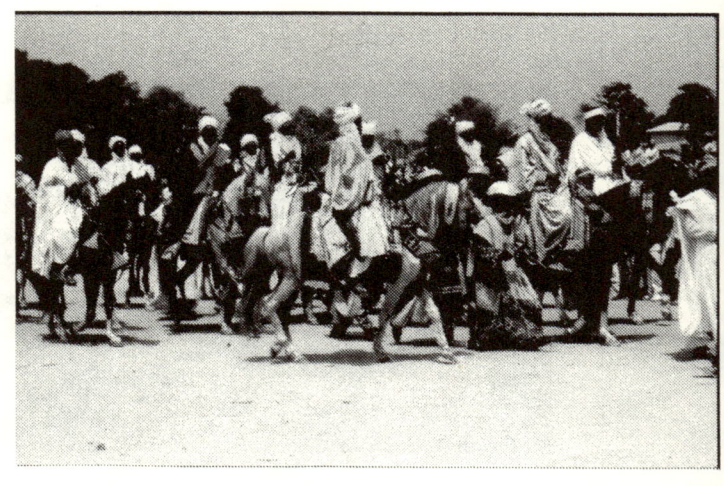

Picture 77: Zaria. The lustrous escort.

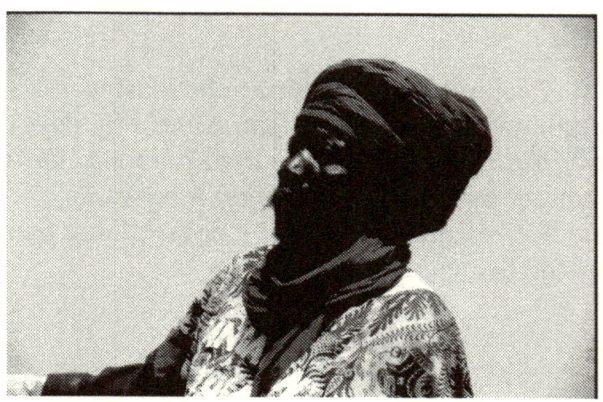

Picture 78: Zaria. One of the Emir's bodyguards.

When the high-ranking dignitaries arrive, the horse race starts.

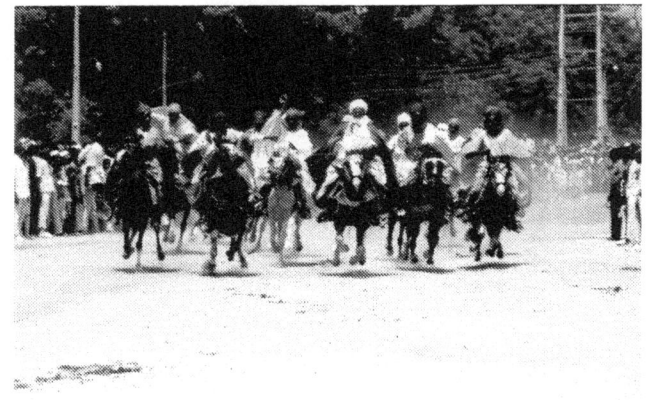

Picture 79: Zaria. Behind the racing horses, dust showers the watching crowd.
These beautiful saddle-horses make up the parade of the nomadic horsemen. Each horse is well decorated and the embroidered costumes of the horsemen are adorned with exquisite silver and fantastic coiled turbans. Truly a colourful fairyland.

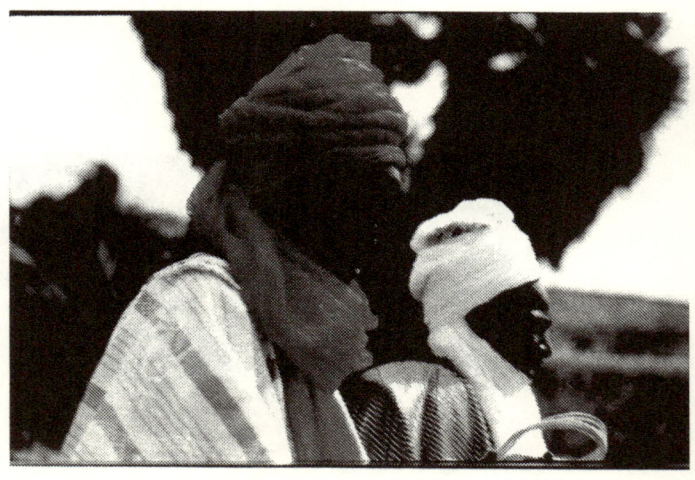

Picture 80: Zaria. The length of the turban material should be 8 metres.

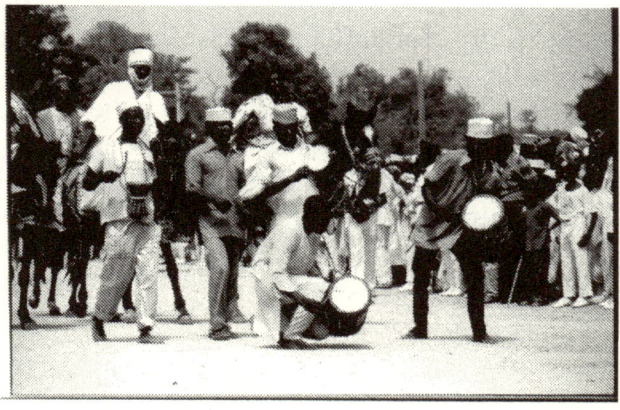

Picture 81: Zaria. A group of drummers
After the horse race, a long line of innumerable groups, dancers and drummers marches before the spectators.

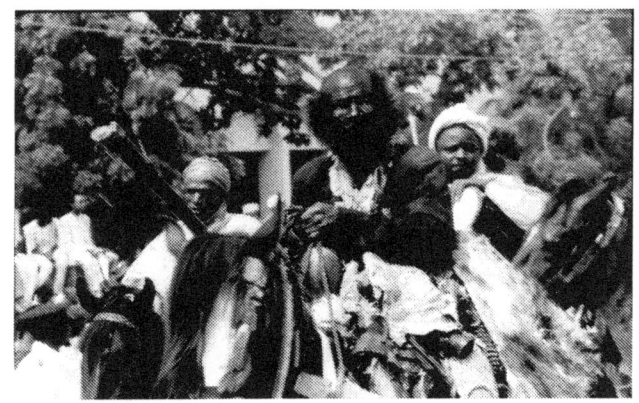

Picture 82: Zaria. The Juju-man.

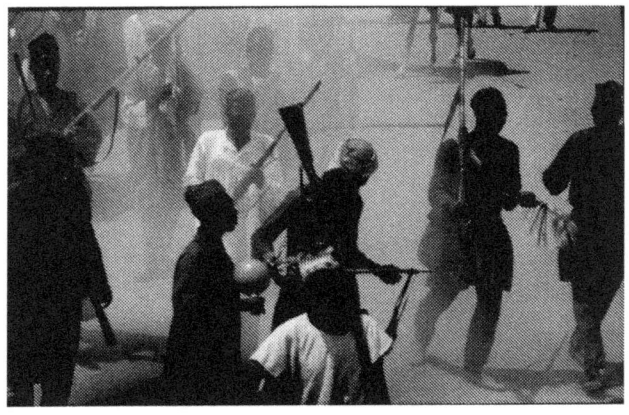

Picture 83: [Enlarge] Zaria. This group is shooting with muzzle-loader guns [a remanent left behind by the

white colonisers of the 18th century], much to the delight of onlookers.
With the ensuing rumpus, lost within the cacophony of the noisy crowd, this was the best time to leave.

EAST AFRICA

THE SUDAN

The Sudan is the largest country in Africa but has a population of only 30 million. After Anglo-Egyptian rule, independence came in 1957, bringing with it a military dictatorship. This was followed by civil war, which brutally ravaged the countryside. Such military violence, lack of consensus and political disorder has been characteristic of this country for a very long time. The war between the north and south of Sudan ended but a few years ago, another war started in Darfur province [North West] again.

Both kidnapping and the slave trade still are active in present-day Sudan. Young boys and girls are taken from their families and are either sold, or end up in an Arab harem.

Despite these problems, the Sudan remains a connecting link between the Arab world and black Africa. Though the agriculture is mostly underdeveloped, irrigated agriculture has long been a prosperous venture between the Blue and White Nile [Gezira Project]. This area, where maize, sugar cane, millet, sesame, groundnuts, rice, cotton, sorghum and gum arabicum [glue base] are all successfully produced, may well secure the future of the country.

The official languages of the country are English and Arabic. About 40 % of the population are Arab and have

mostly lived around the capital and in the north for generations.
Aside from the Arabs, the most well known indigenous tribes are the Nuer, Nubian, Bea, Nubba, Fur, Shilluk, Dinka and Djali. These groups are generally curly haired with very dark, almost bluish black skin [Negroid].
The capital of the Sudan is Khartoum.

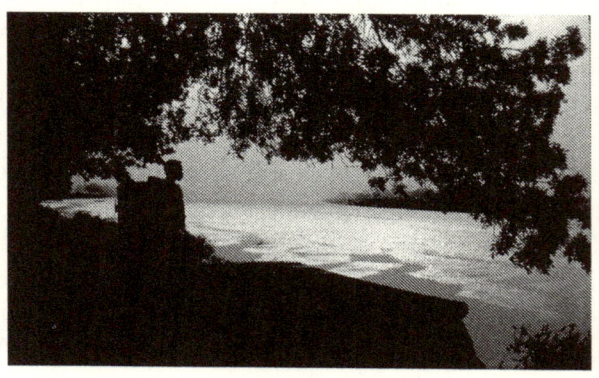

Picture   84: The River Nile covered by the dust of the Habub in Khartoum around midday.
There is frequent exposure to the Saharan dust winds [Habub], which cover everything with its destructive force.

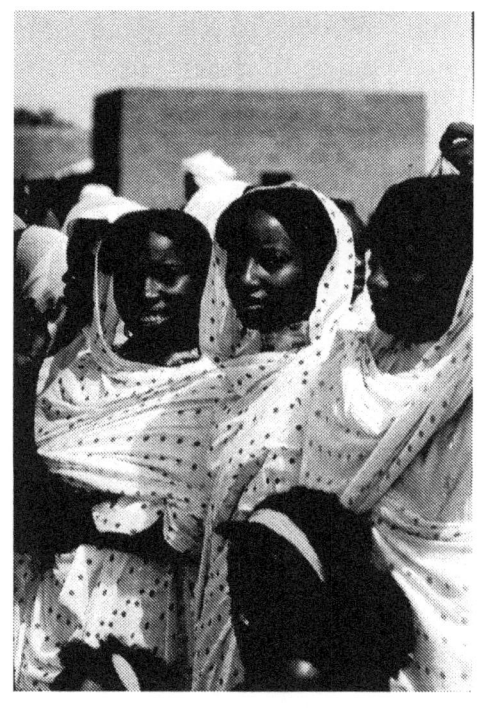

Picture   85:   Arab girls in Nyala.

The Sahel-zone
Stretching south from the Sahara is the Sahel-zone, covering many thousands of miles from the Atlantic coast down to the Red Sea. It is also called the hunger zone. Lack of rain, drought and water shortages characterise this region. As the climate is unfortunately changing towards the south, larger and larger areas are becoming unproductive.
In these huge areas [e.g. northern Sudan and Ethiopia], long droughts and famine are all too common.

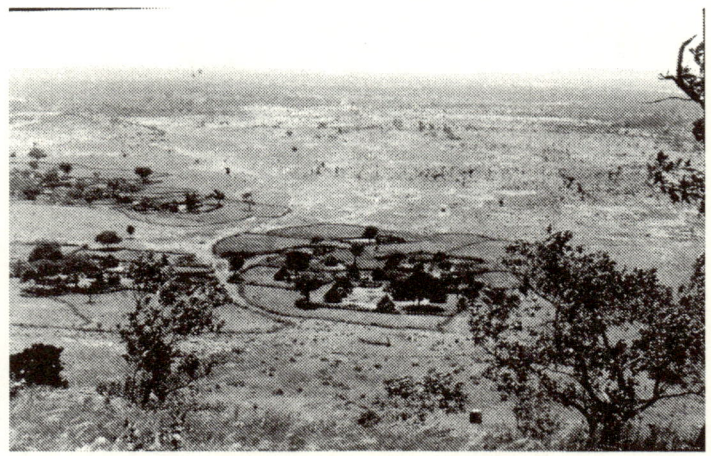

Picture 86: North-West- Sudan. The round grass huts scattered on the savannah blend into the horizon.

More than half of Sudan falls within the Sahel zone. The life of the people living in this vast area is uncertain because the success of their crops depends entirely on the unpredictable rains.

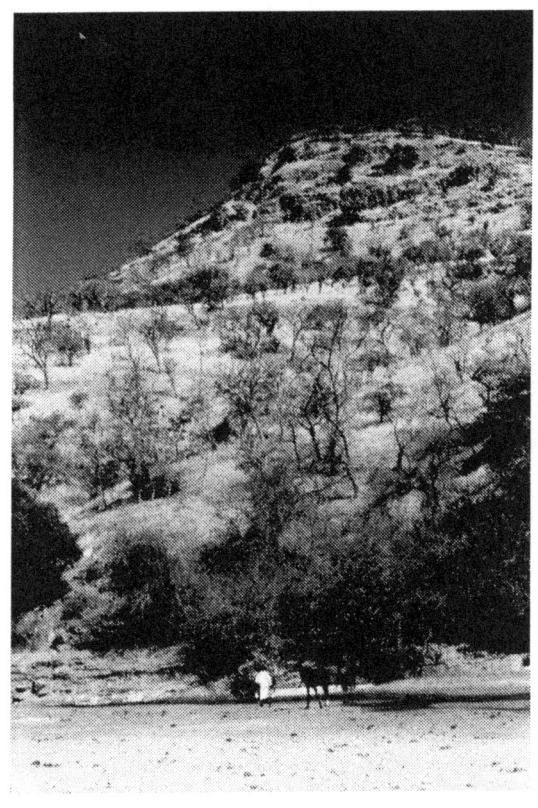

Picture 87: Darfur area. Wadi Azum in the dry season.

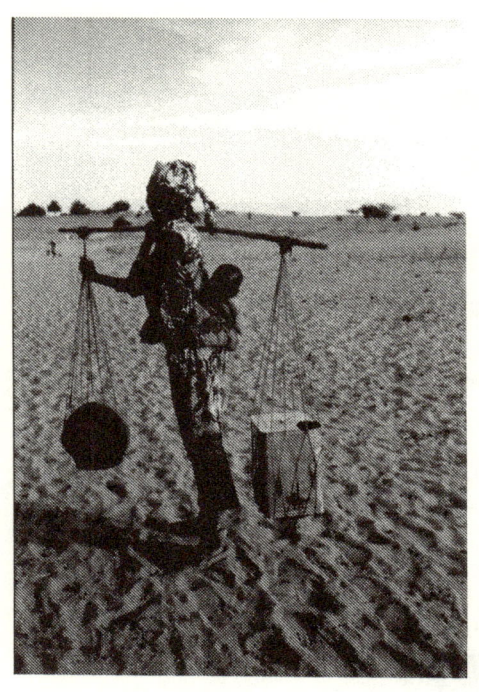

Picture 88: North West, Sudan.
Every day, the women have to walk for miles to collect water.

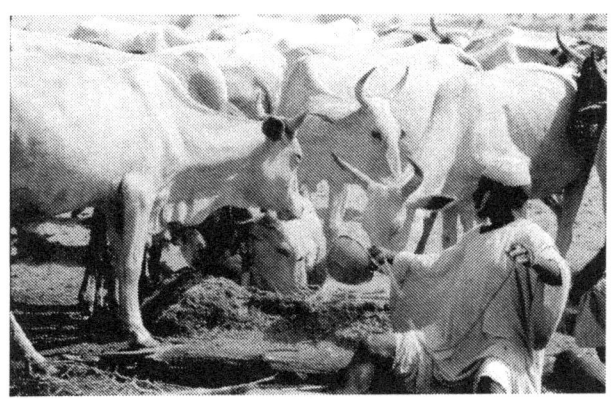

Picture 89: North West, Sudan. Watering the cattle is a very slow process.

The main character trait of the indigenous people is their ingenuity, possessing as they do, an amazing ability to adapt to the desolate environment. They have lived a nomadic migrating life from time immemorial.

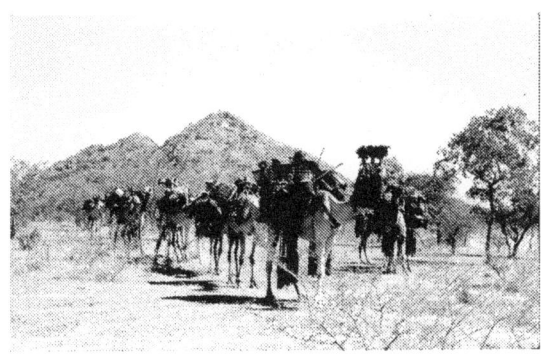

Picture 90: Darfur territory. Camel caravan approaches the Wadi Azum.

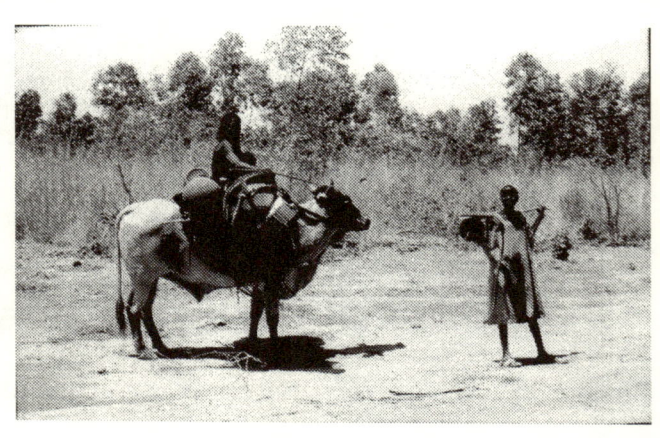

Picture 91: Darfur territory. Migrating Rezeqat family. All belongings are loaded at the side.

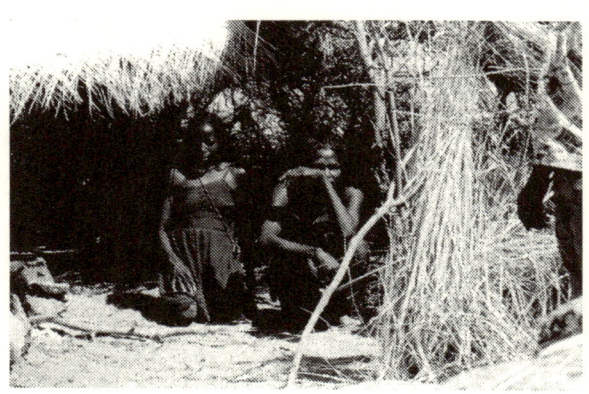

Picture 92: North West. Even today, some of the minor tribe are completely isolated from the rest of the world.

Nowadays, old traditions are slowly fading away. More and more people are starting to settle in villages and are learning agriculture.

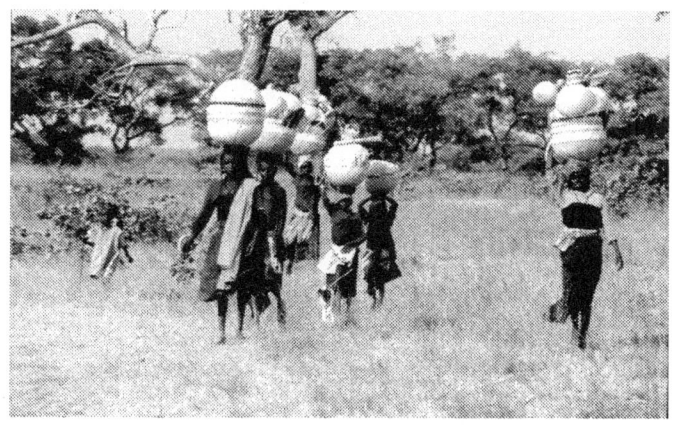

Picture 93 : Darfur area. Women on their long journey to the local market.

The wife of the nomadic herdsman has to walk long miles to the closest village market in order to sell milk or home-made cheese. She carries her child on her back and the goods on her head. The weight-bearing capacity of the women is enormous. The great loads on their heads are carried with a straight back and a sure foot.

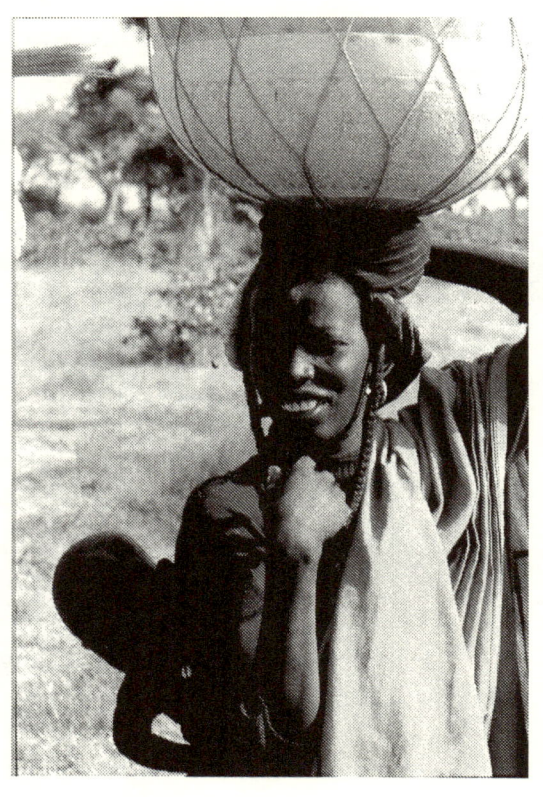

Picture 94: She is going to the Zalingei market.

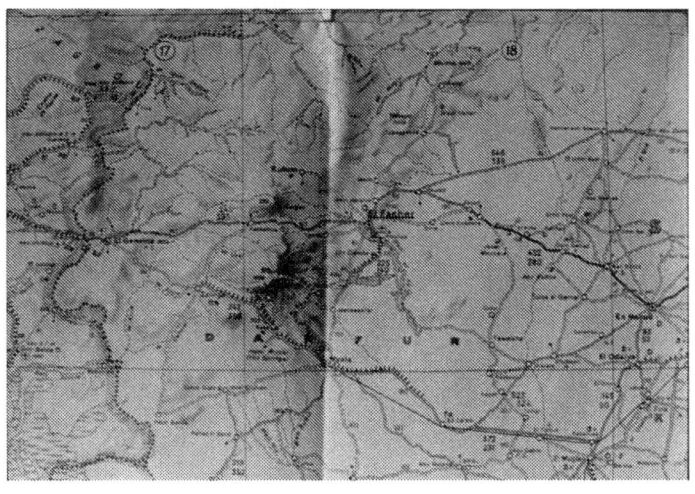

The map of Darfur area – Sudan.

Darfur province

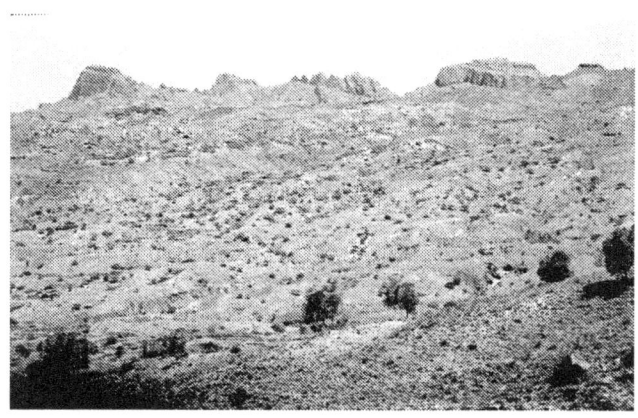

Picture 95: Jabel Marra – Darfur.
The romantic Jebel Marra mountain is situated in the west of the country, its foothills extending to the savannah. Leopard and wild ass roam the area.

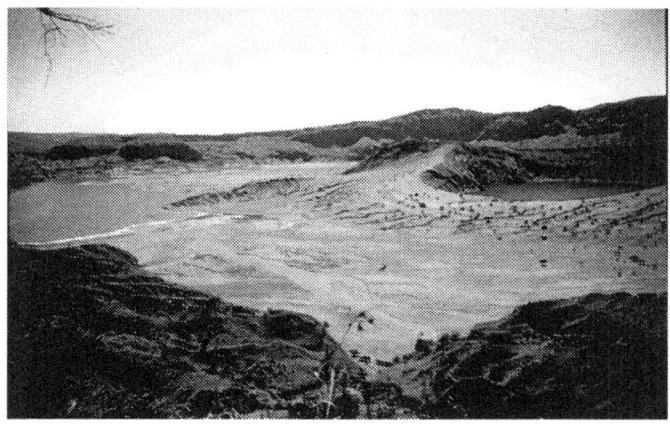

Picture 96: The crater of Jabel Marra.

In the great crater of this volcanic mountain, about 8 kms in diameter, is a salt-water lake. During the slow geological development within the crater, a smaller, secondary crater was also formed, which is a glistening fresh-water mountain lake.
According to the beliefs of the local populace, an evil demon resides in the fresh-water lake, who mercilessly drags down anyone who dares to bathe there. In the salt-water lake, however, a good spirit resides, allowing anyone to bathe in its water.

In and around the area of Jebel Marra [Darfur] live the Fur ethnic groups. The Fur are settled, peaceful and hardworking farming people.

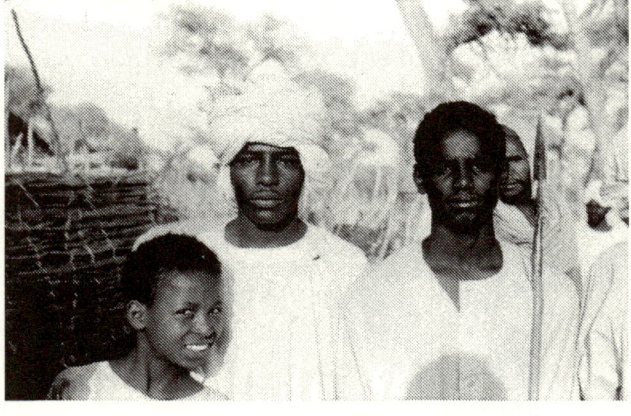

Picture 97: The young of the Fur who inhabit the Nyertete village.

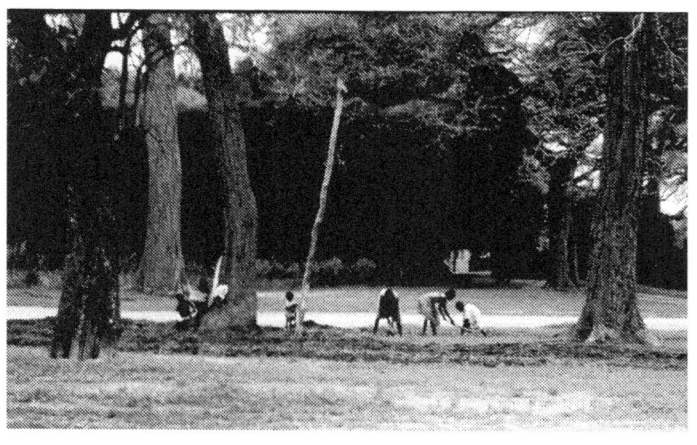

Picture: 98: Zalingei. Cultivating the land is always hard work. In the upper region, water is plentiful and here they grow fruit and vegetables. On the flat lowlands, the crops are sorghum, millet, sesame and groundnuts. But today, no one knows what is going on there, because of the war.

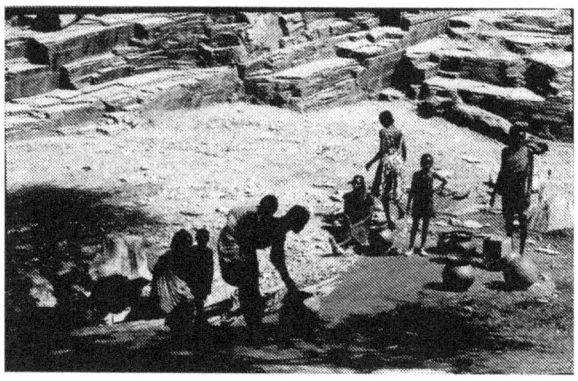

Picture   99:   Near Zalingei. Water-hole.
It is the women's work to bring the water supply for the day. In the dry season, water is scarce and has to be brought in from a great distance. The sizeable earthenware containers are slowly filled from dug wells and carried home on their heads.

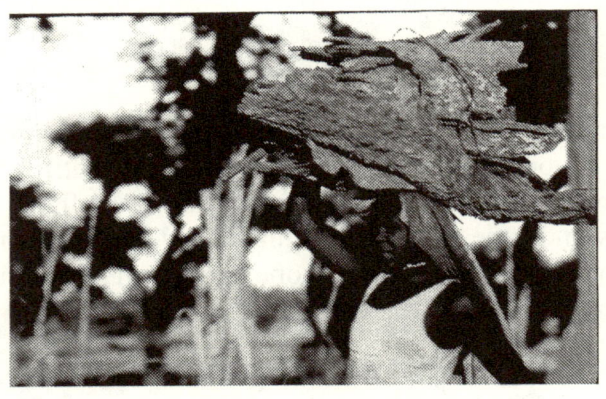

Picture   100:   Zalingei.
Collecting firewood is also women's work. They frequently carry large loads on their heads. This probably explains why the posture of African women is so beautifully balanced.

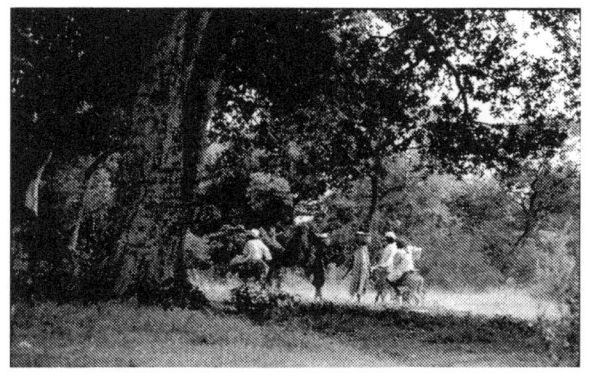

Picture 101: Nyertete. On the way home from market. Donkeys are a popular domestic animal, but unfortunately, most of the time they are grossly overloaded.

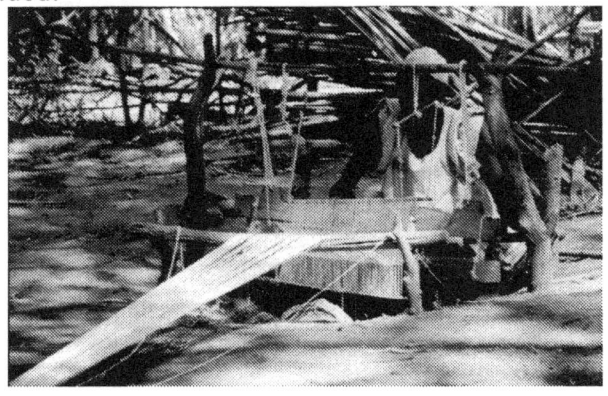

Picture 102: Primitive loom in Umbala village.

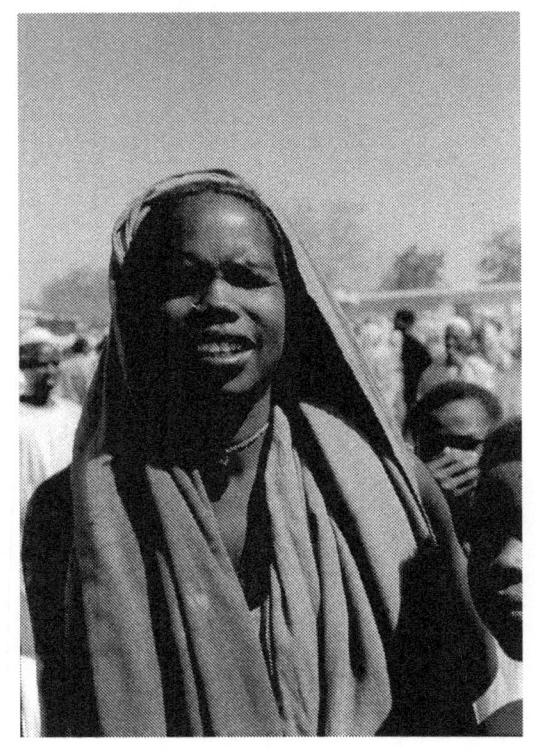

Picture   103:   Fur woman in Nyala.

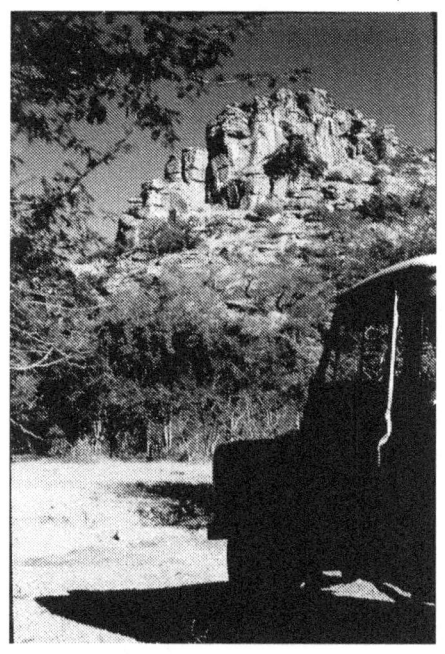

Picture 104: Darfur territory. A picturesque mountain top in the Marra foot hills.

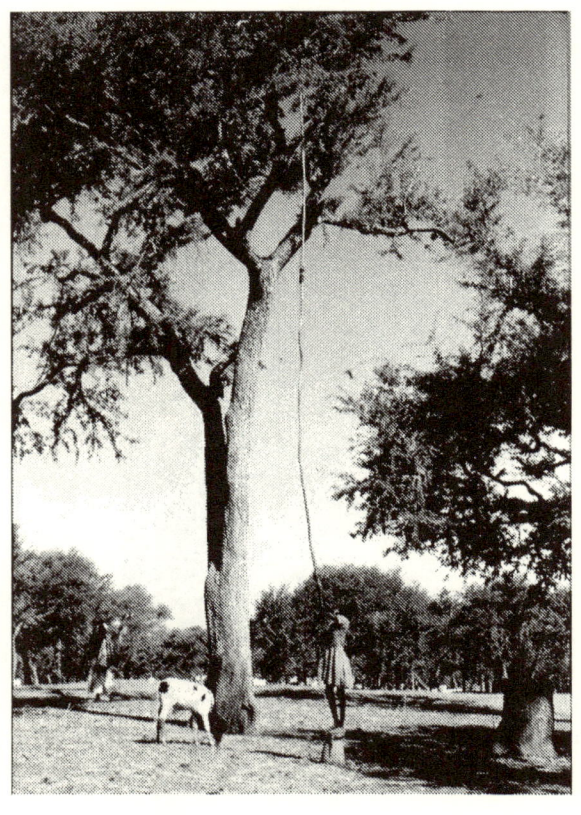

Picture 105: Zalingei. Ingenious tool to harvest seed pods from tall trees.

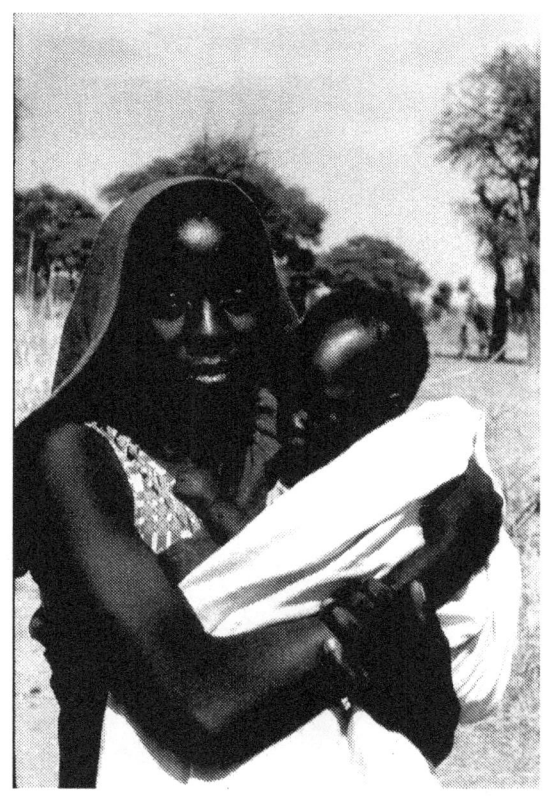

Picture 106: Mother and child in the Fur inhabited village of Zalingei.

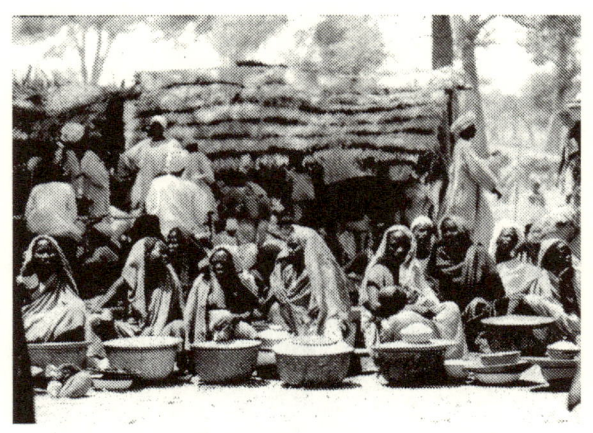

Picture 107: Zalingei. The Fur women are slim and usually cover themselves with soft, light blue folded materials. They go to the local markets in groups and sell their goods together.

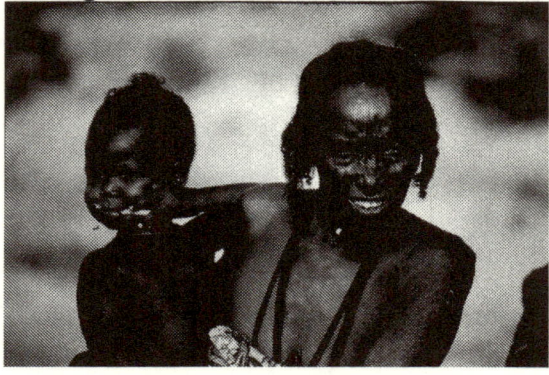

Picture 108: Rural woman with her child in Zalingei.

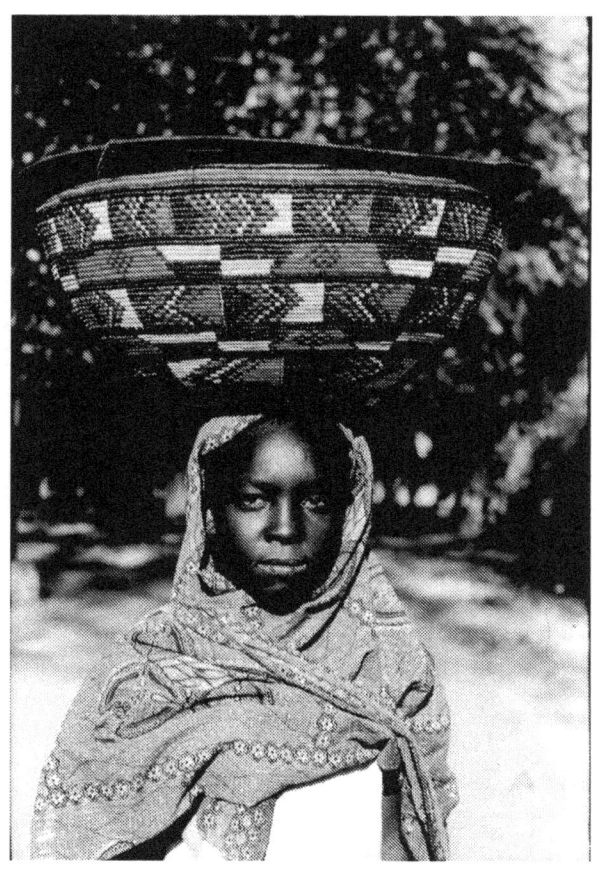

Picture 109 : Zalingei. Sudanese basket weaving is of an outstanding quality. The colour red is often used and intricate patterns are commonplace.

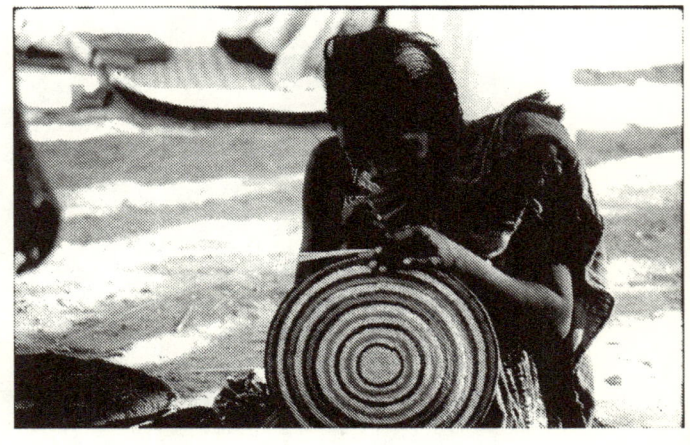

Picture 110: Zalingei. From grass, the skilled women make beautifully patterned plates, baskets and even vessels for carrying milk. The latter are so closely woven that curiously enough, the milk cannot escape through the wall of the vessel. They are never washed.

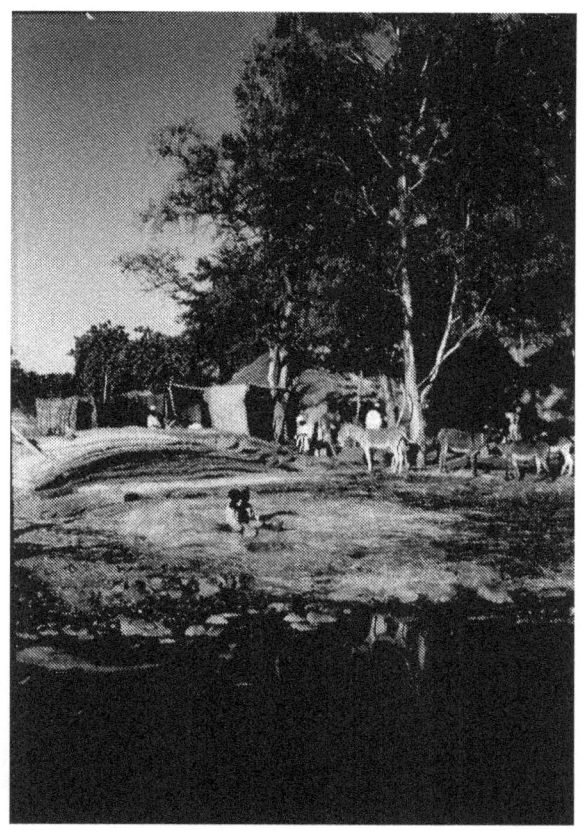

Picture 111: Nyertete. A peaceful evening time.

Today, in Darfur province, a peaceful evening time is just a dream. Nowadays everything has changed for the worse due to the war. In the hands of the bush soldiers, modern weapons glisten under the hot rays of the sun and the firing of shots is merciless. Life is cheap here.

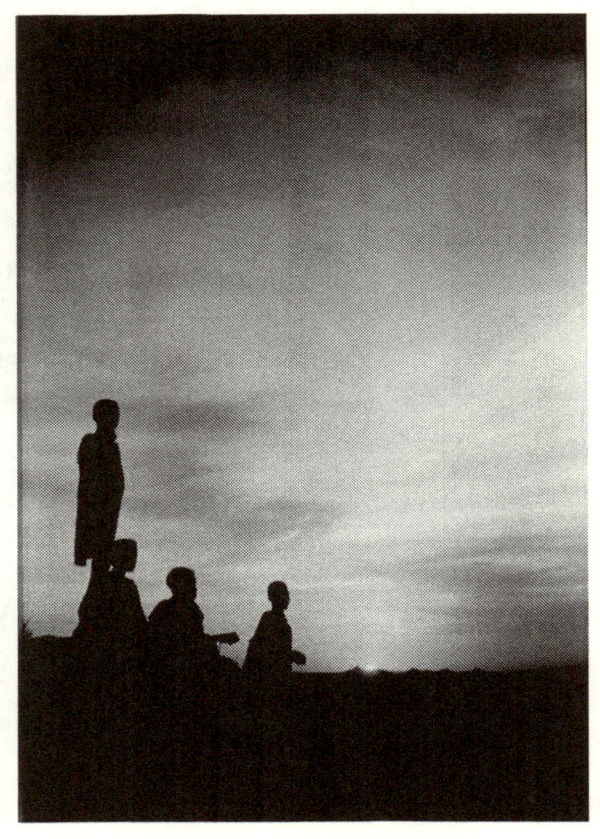

Picture 112: Sunset in Darfur.

DISEASE

In most areas of Africa, the surface water is contaminated and not suitable for direct consumption. Nevertheless, with no other option, the people have to drink it all the same.
It is not advisable to bathe in the slow-flowing waters and lakes, due to the risk of bilharzia infection, spread by water snails which act as carriers. When the ensuing infection sets in and the intestinal parasites get a grip, the abdomen swells up.

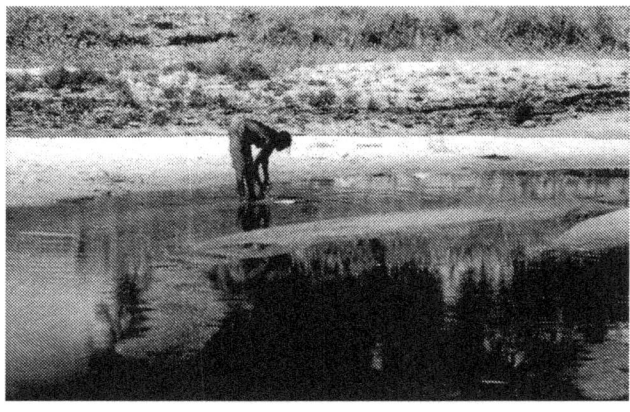

Picture 113: Wadi Azum – Darfur territory – The Sudan.. Fur woman washing her dress. This is a common sight all over Africa.

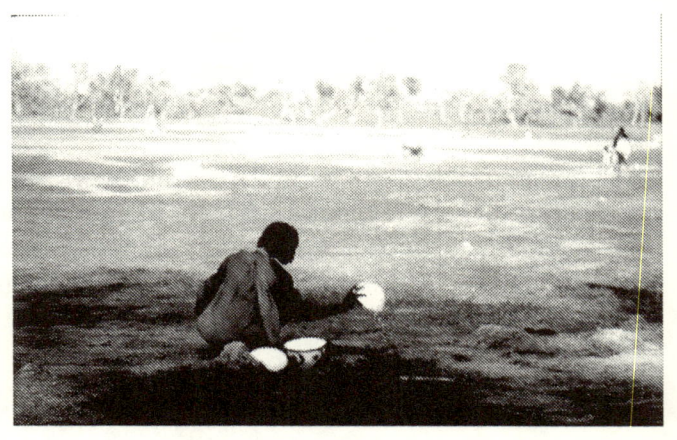

Picture 114: Wadi-Azum- Darfur territory – The Sudan. Drinking water is collected from the river bed.

Children die every day from diarrhoea, which is a disease caused by infected water.

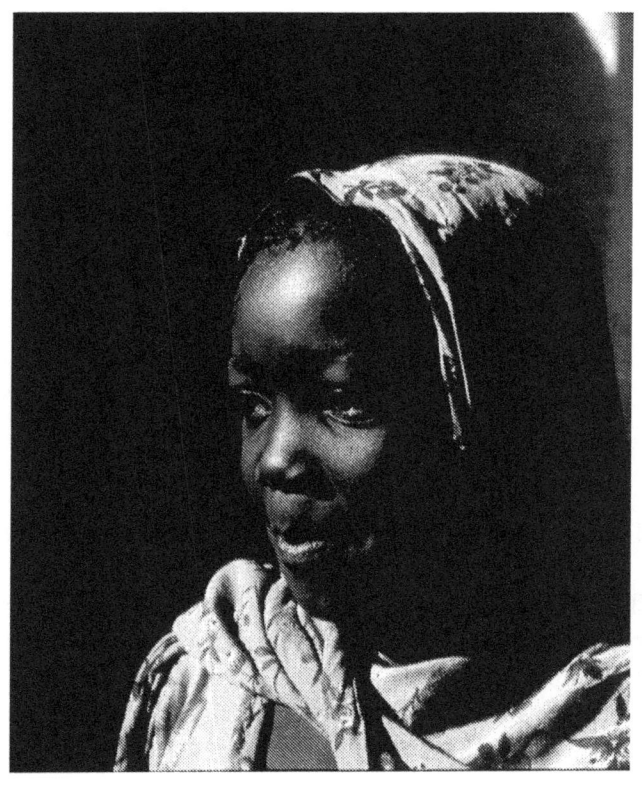

Picture 115: Young girl from Nyala – The Sudan.

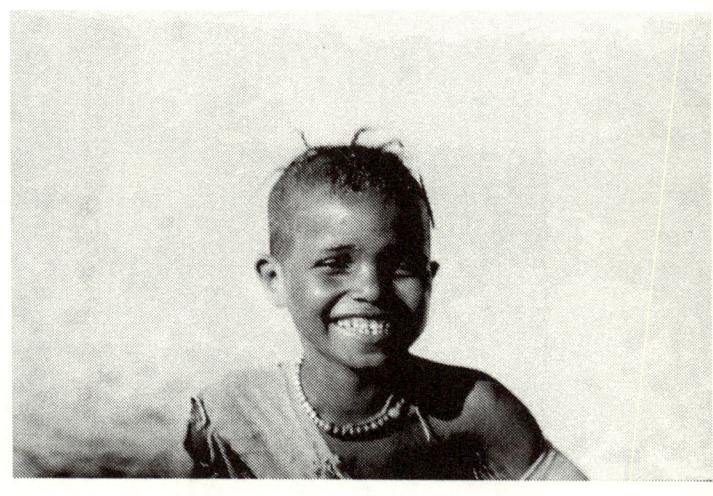

Picture 116: Little Fur child in Zalingei – The Sudan.

The tropical climate, the heat, the small insects, the mosquitoes and the flies all increase the risk of infection.
In the suburbs and markets, the black, stinking sewage flows freely between the alleyways. Beside the roads, children sift through the rubbish heaps.
In the overcrowded cities, public sanitation is inadequate, and the same is true of the countryside. There are not enough doctors, medicine, equipment, and the water is usually not sanitised.
Diseases such as malaria, yellow fever, sleeping sickness, cholera, river blindness, and most recently HIV/AIDS, are all widespread.

Trying to combat these contagious diseases has long been a difficult task. This is a problem which will not go away.

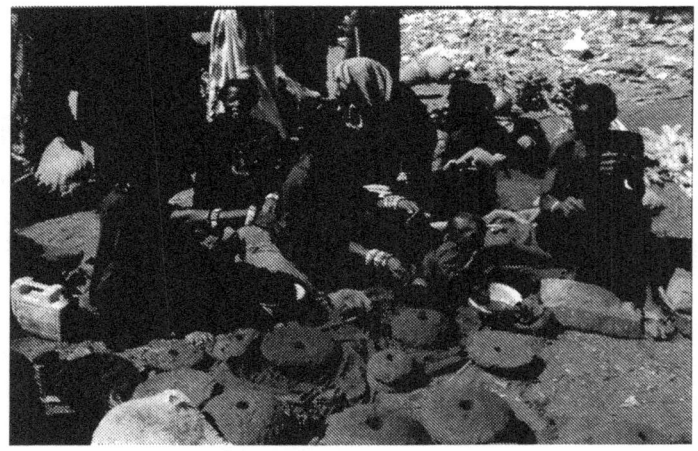

Picture 117: South Niger. Rubbish is everywhere in the market.
The majority of people are uneducated and unaware of the effect of poor hygiene.

Villagers are strongly superstitious. Many believe that if someone dies, the spirit will move into the body of one of the snakes living around the house. If someone is bitten by a snake, it means that one of the ancestors is angry with him or her. There can be no escape. This person is doomed to death. In most cases, relatives don't even bother calling a doctor. Instead, rural people tend to turn to witch-doctors.

The juju-man cures with a mixture of magic, incantations and herbal concoctions in order to drive out the evil spirits. Quite simply, the patient will either die or recover.

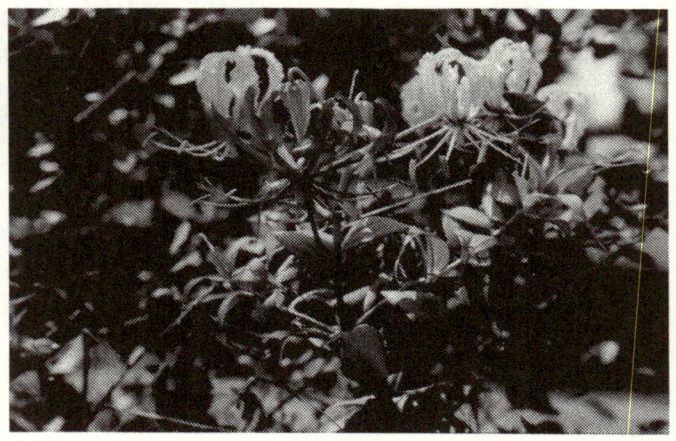

Picture   118:   Climbing lily [Glorious lily] in the bush. Its tuber is used as medicine.

THE VOICE OF AFRICA

Africa manages to mirror the past, present and future all at the same time.
During the past century, many African countries gained independence, but this has usually meant civil war or confrontation from outside. The effects of this are still felt today, with a constant struggle for power, mixed with corruption and confusion.

It is no secret that millions are born into poverty every day. Although the death rate is high, the population in the western parts of Africa has doubled, with more than half of the populace under the age of 15. However, countless women die in childbirth. Information about birth control is limited and this is as yet an unsolved problem.

Some governments of African countries are starting to invest large sums of money into information services and education. Despite this, the number of illiterate is still high.

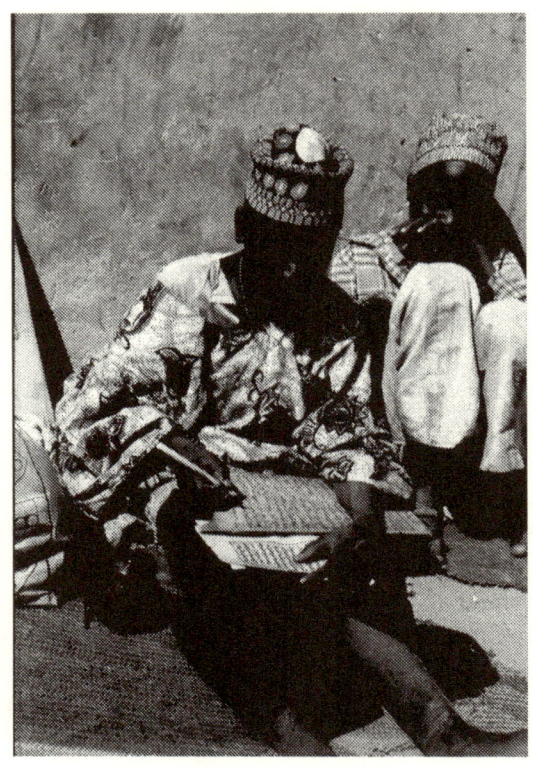

Picture 119: Zaria - Nigeria. Schoolboys.

Many children still do not attend school regularly. In Islamic regions, it is common to cram only the Holy Koran into the pupil's head. However, it is very important to give children a quality education.

Famine and finding water in the dry season are the biggest problems throughout the Sahel zone.

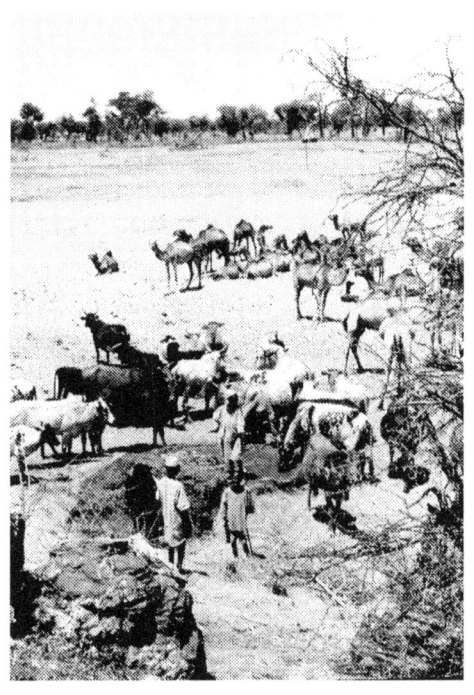

Picture 120: Darfur region – Sudan. Thirsty herd in the dry river bed.

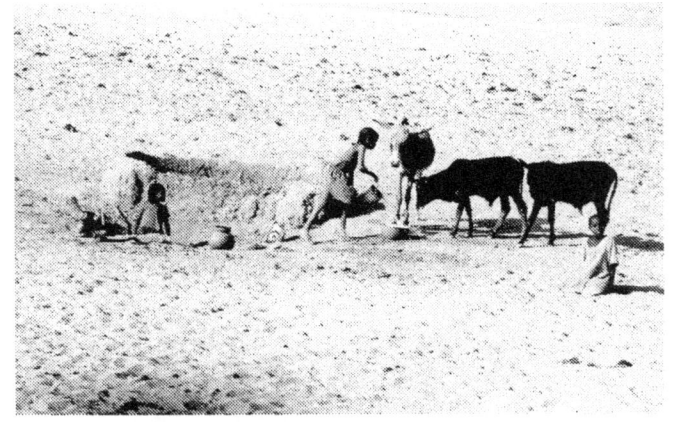

Picture 121: Darfur area – the Sudan. Children learn to value water from an early age, and under the hot sun they are working too.

In rural areas, markets represent the only opportunity to make cash.

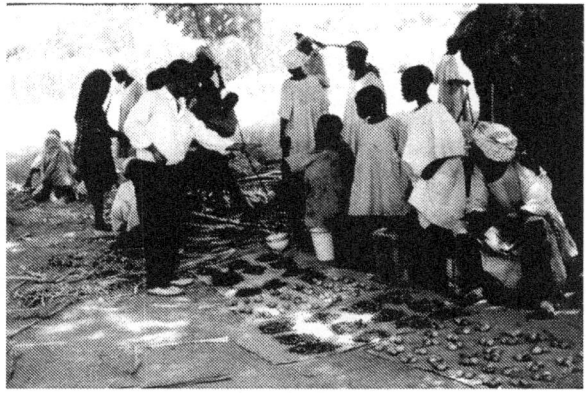

Picture 122: Between Umbala and Zalingei – the Sudan. Shopping in the market.

The image of poverty is everywhere.

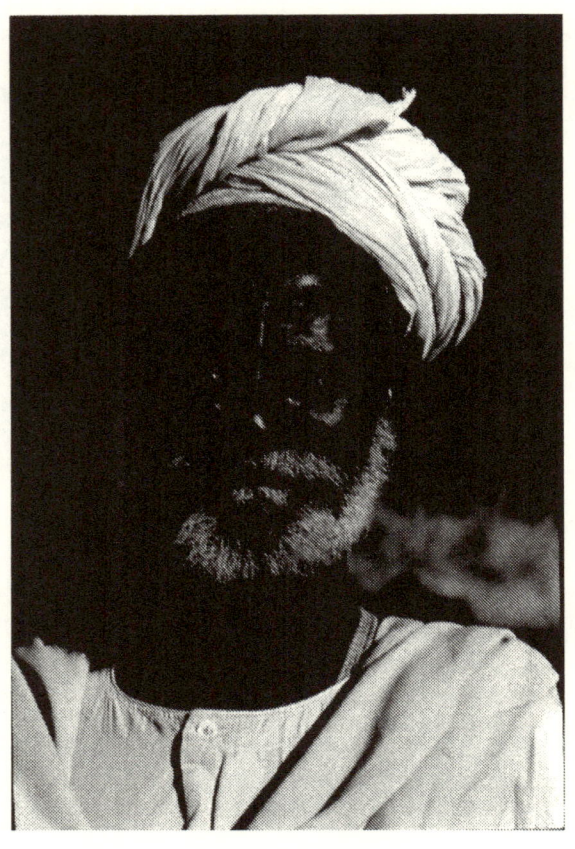

Picture 123: Nyala –Sudan. An old man who said he has no opportunity for a better life.

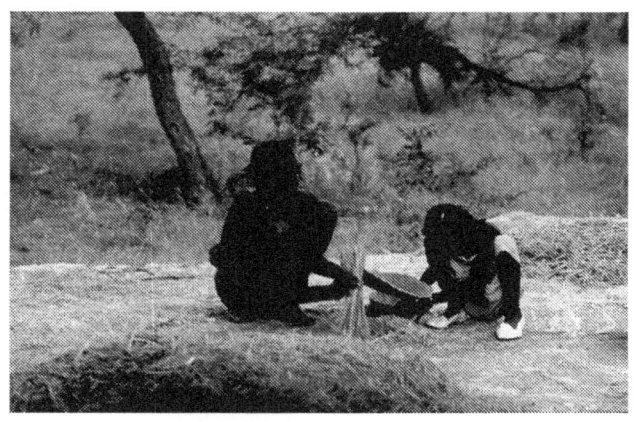

Picture 124: Nyertete – Sudan. The most poverty-stricken collect grass seeds. This is also a way of getting food.

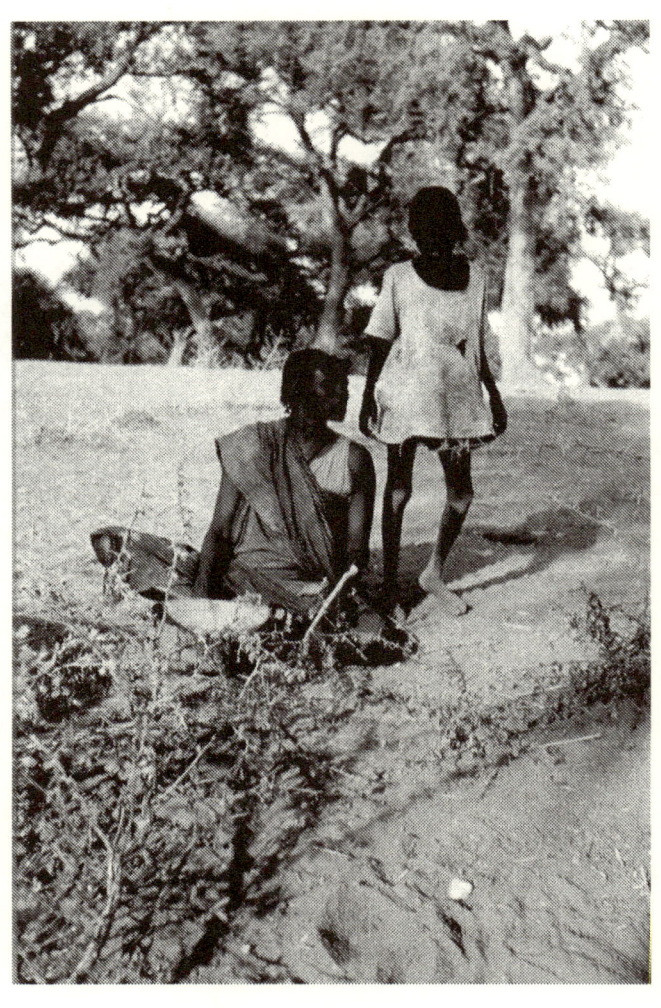

Picture 125: Zalingei – Sudan. A Fur woman collects acacia-albaida pods for fodder.

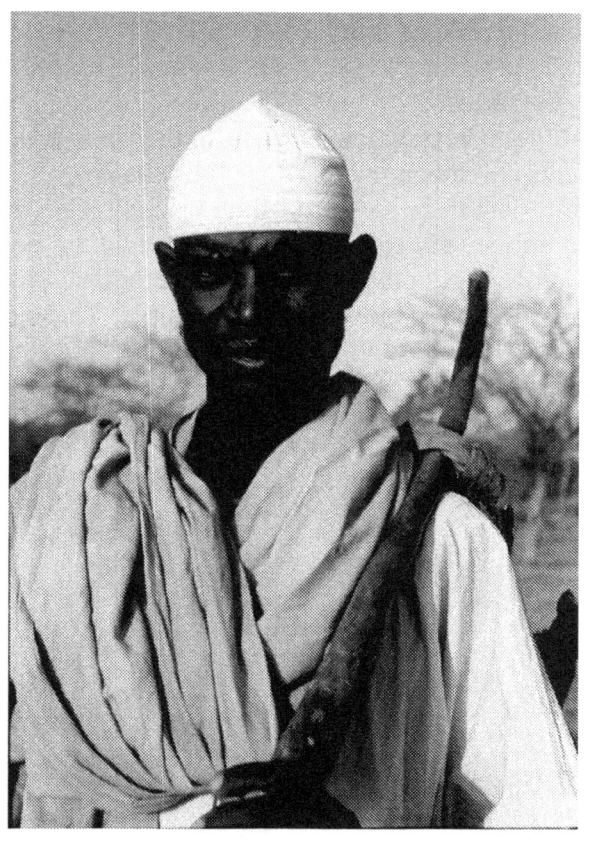

Picture 126: Nyertete – Sudan. Fur man.

The development of industry and agriculture in Africa is rather slow. Natural conditions in most countries are favourable but without adequate machinery, quality

seeds and expertise, the farmers are not able to achieve results and without help, it is not possible for them to even get started.
Probably the best way forward is to devise a programme and send volunteers who are well-educated agriculturists from any part of the world. If they were to stay a number of years, they could educate the people about more productive agricultural methods and set up as many demonstration farms as possible. These projects should be ongoing with no fixed end-date and financed by the assisting organisations.

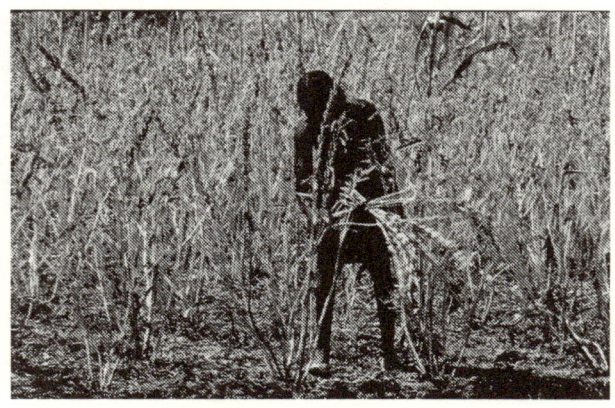

Picture 127: Umbala –Sudan. Sesame harvest.

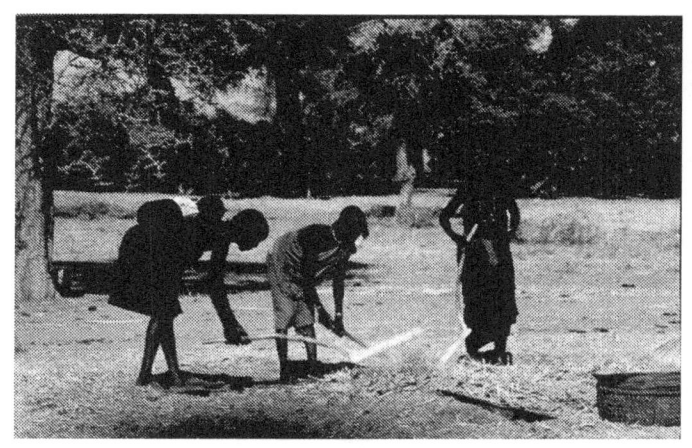

Picture 128: Zalingei – Sudan. Threshing is women's work.

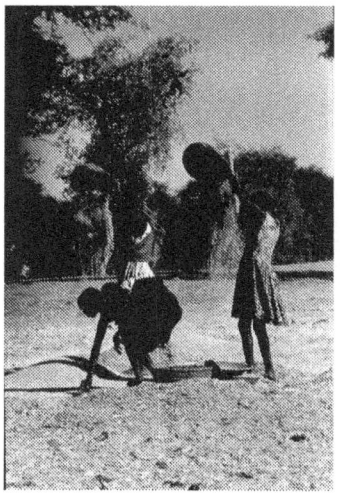

Picture 129: Zalingei – Sudan. Winnowing.

In a few countries [e.g. Kenya], however, agriculture is developing quickly. Good results have also been achieved in some parts of Nigeria, which proves that with committed, disciplined work and expert help, food production can be increased.

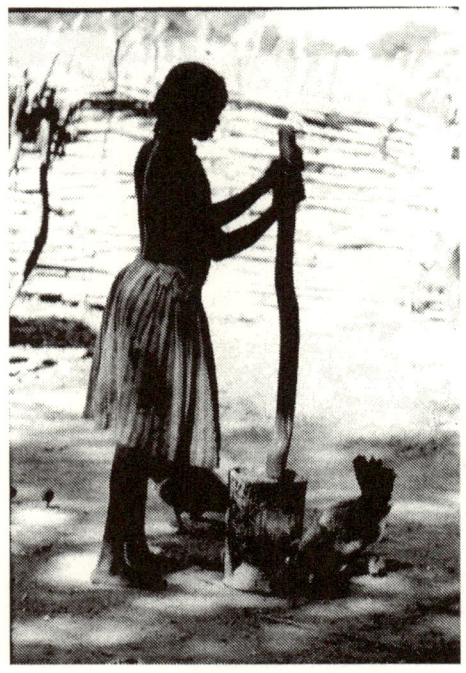

Picture 130: Darfur region – Sudan. Woman grinding millet.

I am well aware that these problems have been publicised many times in the past but not enough has been done because poverty, lack of clean water, famine and disease still predominate in Africa. There is no need to explain that the basic problems, even today, have changed little.

It is difficult to find a solution and even large international organisations have failed to come up with one so far. They do help a lot, but this is only a drop in the ocean. They send money, food, many kinds of goods, medication, clothes, and so on. However this kind of help is not always the best and does not represent the most effective long-term solution because the bulk of the consignments often simply disappear [e.g. Ethiopia and the Sudan], while at the same time famine spreads uncontrollably. The foodstuffs, grains etc. often simply end up in the hands of well-connected traders who sell it on the markets for their own profit.

Remember the story about fishing. Better to teach how to fish than hand out free fish.

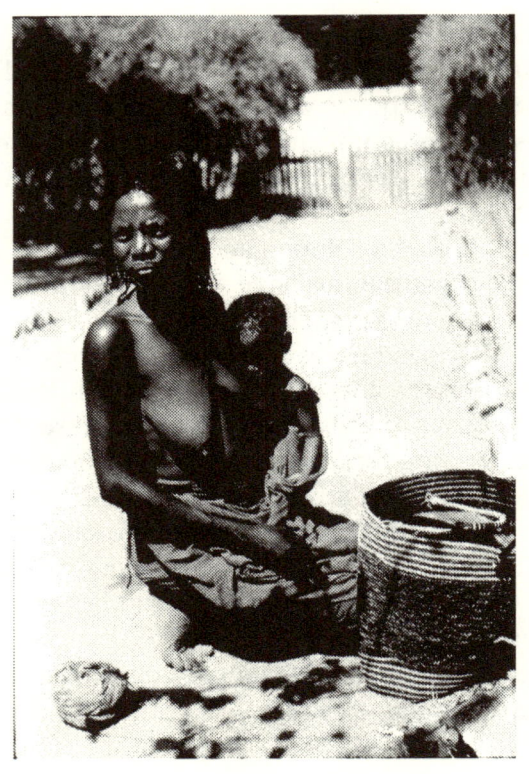

Picture 131: Zalingei – Sudan. No comment.

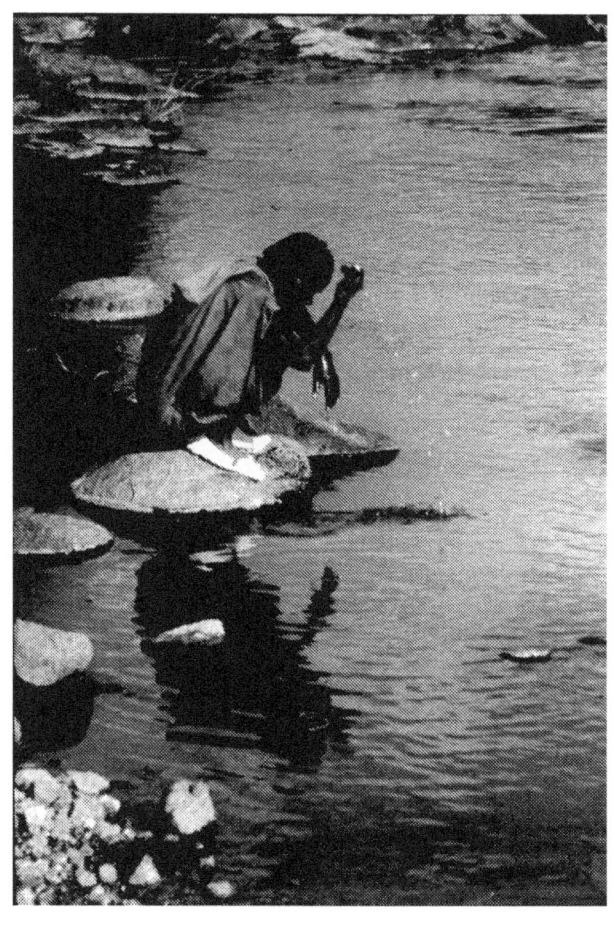

Picture 132:   Nyertete – Sudan. Day dreaming.

I believe that soon, many African people will feel the need to stand up. To stand up alone, empowered with peace, new knowledge, skills and techniques.

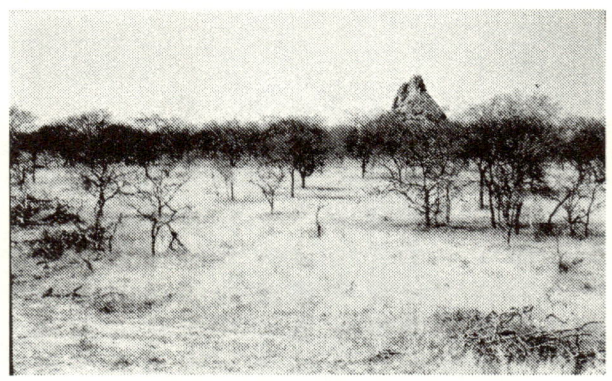

Picture 133: West Sudan. The wonderful landscape.

KENYA
The Eden of Africa

Africa is a continent where one can still find nature's untouched harmony. The colourful culture of the indigenous tribes and the awe-inspiring wildlife both deserve a special place within the continent's natural and cultural heritage.

Anyone who has ever visited Africa will find it hard to forget the passing of gnu herds on the distant horizon, the bouncing of gazelles, the rush of chased animals through trembling air, the harmony and speed of the cheetah.
One can feel fear and admiration at the same time.
When I first caught sight of the snow-covered peak of Mount Kilimanjaro (Kabo) and the slow movement of animals through the surrounding savannah, I truly felt as if I were in Eden.

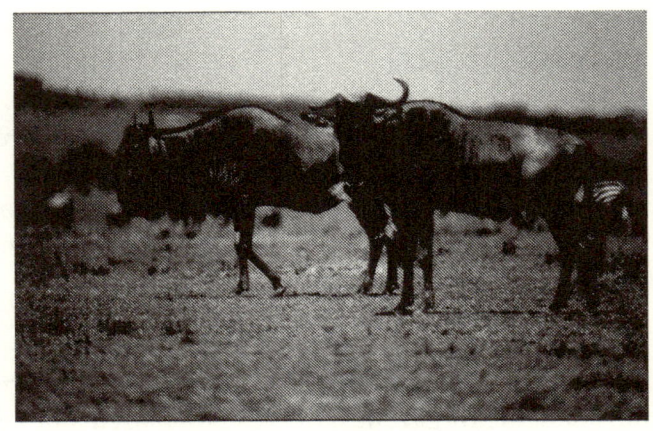

Picture 134: Amboseli National Park –Kenya. Migrating gnus.

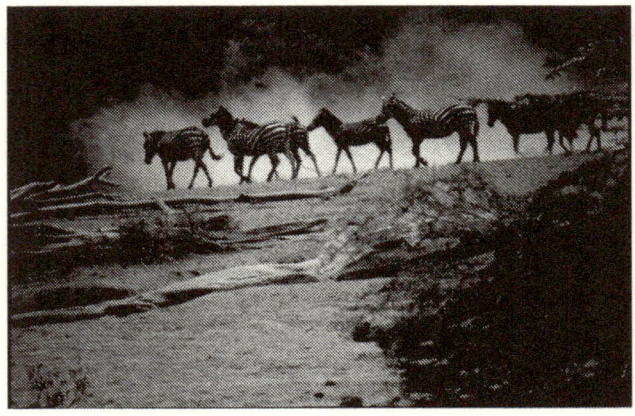

Picture 135: Tsavo West National Park – Kenya. The slow movement of Zebras.

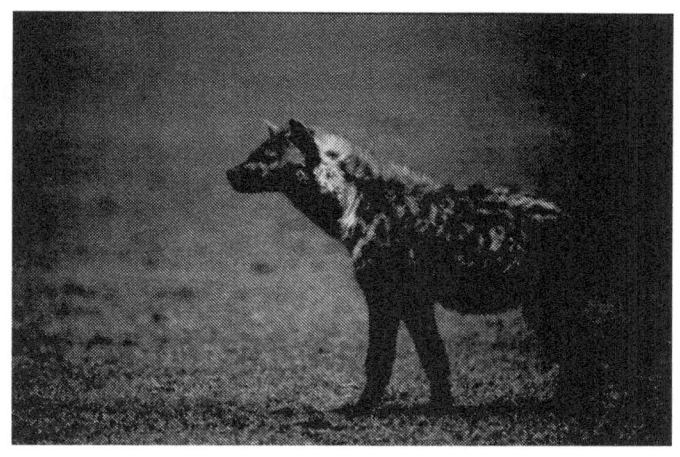

Picture 136: Masai Mara – Kenya. Young hyena hunting for prey.

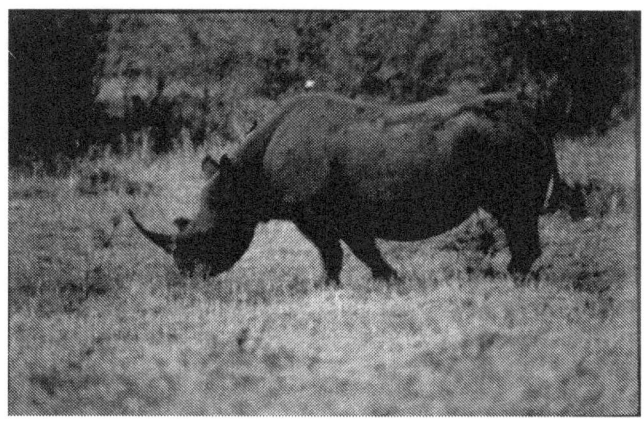

Picture 137: Amboseli National Park – Kenya. Rhino is one of the big five.

I can still see the stony stare of the rhino. I am still enthralled by the menacing movement of lions around our car. They were so close to us. I remember when our driver suddenly pulled up the car window due to the presence of the lions. Ten minutes later, back in the camp, the windows wouldn't budge any more and this was compounded by a flat tyre. I still shiver when I think what the outcome might have been if this had happened a few minutes earlier.

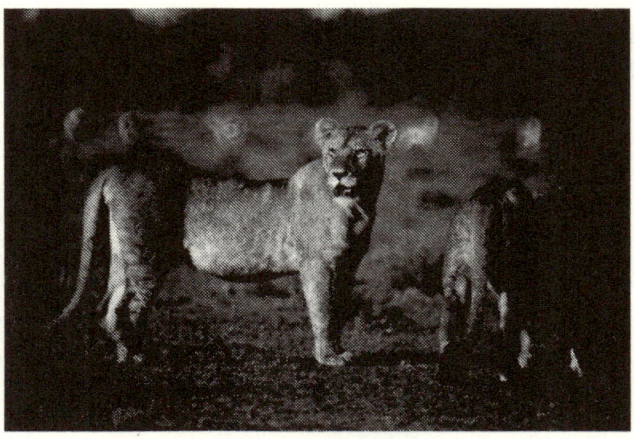

Picture 138: Fig Tree Camp – Kenya. Lions prepare for the early morning hunt.

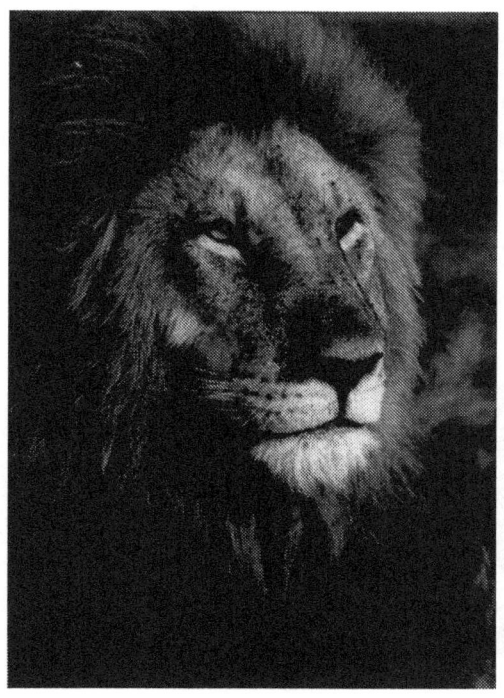

Picture 139: Fig Tree Camp – Kenya. In the background, the lion kept an eye on the nearby grazing gazelles for a short time and then turned its attention to our car.

I can still taste the fear I felt when the buffalo attacked our car during a safari. Fortunately, our driver was very skilled and drove in a zigzag pattern, enabling us to escape.

The thrill of adventure, mingled with excitement and fear, provides an experience unique to this continent.

However, the future of the existing wildlife in the National Parks is uncertain.
Game trading, poaching, burning of the savannah, increasing population numbers and in some countries civil war, mean that extinction threatens more and more species.

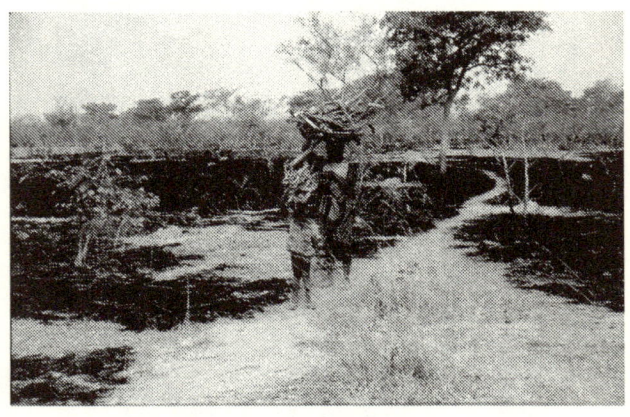

Picture 140: Nigeria. The burnt down area of the Yankari National Park.
The game population in West Africa has almost practically died out.

In Kenya and South Africa, well-run game reserves have been operating for a long time. Here, the preservation and protection of the different species is deliberate. Nowadays, more and more nature conservationists work on the principle that instead of culling elephants or other game populations, they should be re-settled to less stressed areas.

Today, the Maasai say that the wild animals are their friends. It is because of the animals that tourists are visiting Kenya in large numbers, and this in turn makes living easier.

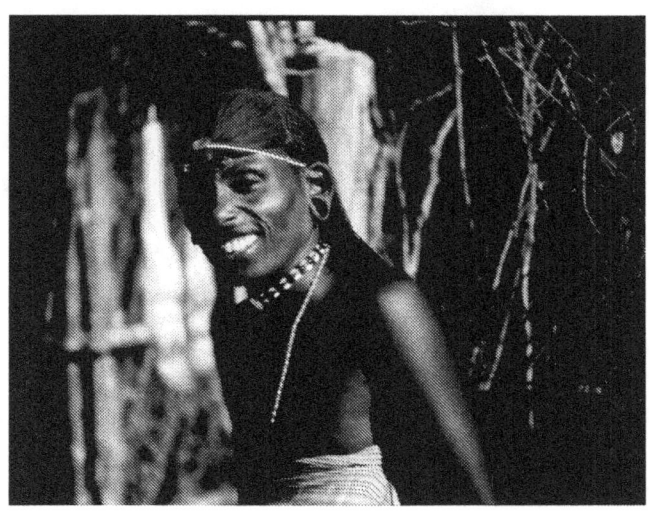

Picture 141:   Masai Mara –Kenya. Maasai man.

This is a continent with so many riches, although the majority of the people do not feel the wealth at their fingertips.
This continent's unique flora and fauna should be saved by all who live there. After all, without these, the true face of Africa will be lost forever.

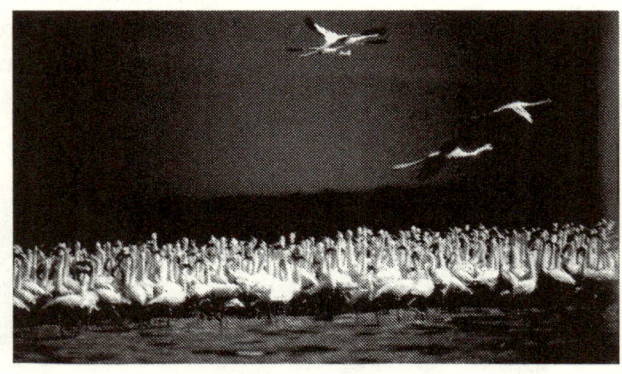

Picture 142: Kenya. Pink flamingos on Lake Nakuru.

Let's preserve this Garden of Eden so future generations can enjoy it as much as we do now.

- When I saw nature's untouched beauty, as present in Africa, I sensed how wonderful the whole world must once have been. And as I thought this, the red disk of the sun slipped over the edge of the horizon and soon darkness covered the land. The stars blinked so close, maybe I could reach up and touch them... –
    -

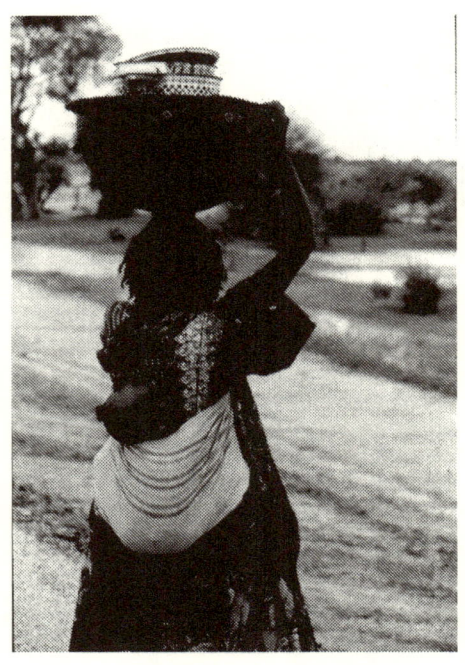

Picture 143: Near Lake Chad – Nigeria. Goodbye Africa, but I will never ever forget you.

Conclusion:

Together, we can all try to help this magnificent continent, which is full of interesting people and exotic wildlife, and together we can try to help protect its natural richness.
Only then we can hope that this living world heritage will remain intact for many future generations to come. Surely, the Africans can learn and choose the best way of progress, doing whatever is needed to be done.
Please do whatever you can to help them reach this state of being.

Thank you.

www.ingramcontent.com/pod-product-compliance
Lightning Source LLC
Chambersburg PA
CBHW020903090426
42736CB00008B/478